Praise for *When Your Child Has Food Allergies*

"Mireille Schwartz openly shares her firsthand experience with and expertise on family food allergies by inviting us to learn and be proactive about food allergies in our communities. As a public health educator and researcher, I appreciate her practical, accessible delivery of information as a key component of creating safe, healthy, and inclusive spaces."

—Evan vanDommelen-Gonzalez, DrPH, MPH

"Mireille Schwartz is a favorite guest on my talk show on KGO810 in San Francisco. My listeners love her and her sensible approach to the challenges of dealing with food allergies. She knows firsthand how difficult this can be since she, her parents, daughter, and brother all have food allergies. Mireille has made it her mission to help others. Let her experience guide you and your family in finding the answers to the frustrating food allergy issues you face."

—Ronn Owens, Talk Radio Host;
inducted into the National Radio Hall of Fame, 2015

"Mireille Schwartz has been educating all of us to the powers of food. We must listen to what this prolific author has to say in her new book When Your Child Has Food Allergies. The hidden allergies that children face can truly make a difference in how they grow up and the deleterious effects that they may carry forward as adults. I'm so excited for this new book, and for all of us to finally become aware of the symptoms and the hidden dangers of allergic reactions."

—Frankie Boyer; Radio Talk Show Host,
"The Frankie Boyer Show"

"Mireille Schwartz provides exemplary food allergy information and insights in an innovative, practical, friendly, and calm style. Decades of her own experience combined with her empathy for others makes for an interesting blend of safe and sane food allergy tips. These are strategies to live by!"

—Jonathan Lawhead, Executive Producer, 2013
Discovery Channel documentary
An Emerging Epidemic: Food Allergies in America

When Your Child Has Food Allergies

When Your Child Has Food Allergies

A PARENT'S GUIDE TO MANAGING IT ALL—
FROM THE EVERYDAY TO THE EXTREME

MIREILLE SCHWARTZ

AMACOM

New York

American Management Association: www.amanet.org
This publication is designed to provide accurate and authoritative information in regard to the subject matter covered. It is sold with the understanding that the publisher is not engaged in rendering legal, accounting, or other professional service. If legal advice or other expert assistance is required, the services of a competent professional person should be sought.

Names: Schwartz, Mireille, 1970– author.
Title: When your child has food allergies : a parent's guide to managing it
  all, from the everyday to the extreme / by Mireille Schwartz.
Description: New York City : American Management Association, [2017]
Identifiers: LCCN 2016048747 (print) | LCCN 2016049673 (ebook) | ISBN
  9780814434055 (pbk.) | ISBN 9780814434062 (ebook)
Subjects: LCSH: Food allergy in children--Treatment--Popular works.
Classification: LCC RJ386.5.S39 2017 (print) | LCC RJ386.5 (ebook) | DDC
  618.92/975--dc23
LC record available at https://lccn.loc.gov/2016048747

10 9 8 7 6 5 4 3 2 1

For
Charlotte Jude,
Dad, Grandmère, and Grandpère

Contents

PART FOUR: Ways You Can Protect Your Child

Introduction

THIS IS A BOOK written by a parent, for parents. So it is full of practical, honest, first hand information about how to cope, and thrive, with a child who has a chronic food allergy. When treating many chronic conditions in children, parents dispense medication but otherwise play a relatively passive role. That's not the case with food allergies. You, as well as all your children and your innermost circle, are responsible for managing the allergy on a daily basis—and will most likely be the first people to respond to an adverse reaction. In this way, you are your child's best resource, and as a food allergy parent, you are most definitely part superhero—who knew?

Once you incorporate the lifestyle changes that are absolutely essential to keeping your child safe, you will be able to keenly spot hidden allergens from a mile away, you will read food labels at lightning speed without missing anything, and—by advocating within your community for your child's safety—you will have stretched and grown in ways you might never have thought possible.

After initially receiving a food allergy diagnosis, things can get really interesting and challenging in your life. A food-allergic child still needs to live richly and experience a wide tapestry of things, like trips to the neighborhood playground, vacations to foreign lands, celebrations of milestones, plus the regular day-to-day moments that are spontaneous and special. But it can be hard to see how on earth this might fit into a family's food-allergic life, which needs to be maintained rigidly, cautiously, with everyone remaining completely vigilant. How can you avoid a life of high-alert stress and instead relax enough to enjoy each moment with your family? And how can you teach your food-allergic child to overcome his or her fears to live fully?

These are all riddles I have worked hard to solve throughout my life. I was born with a potentially life-threatening allergy to fish—all fish—and I had to find ways to adapt in an era before there was any awareness or support, when there was no practical education readily available in all doctors' waiting rooms and on so many websites and blogs. And I'll tell you, it was harrowing. There was nothing to guide me except logic. Once I learned that it was possible to train myself to make the most logical deductions, I realized that I could relax and trust my response when a snap decision needed to be made. I found, over and over again, that I was able to unlock the most sensible solution to any food allergy dilemma. And many of these strategies naturally transferred to my role as the parent of a severely nut-allergic daughter.

This book is filled with the logical solutions and ever-ready mentalities that I developed and now want to share. And I also want to reach out, from one parent to another, to bolster your strength as you navigate the myriad challenges that come from your child's allergy. That's why I want to begin this book by sharing the personal story of how the Golden Gate Bridge over the San Francisco Bay became a symbol of living with food allergies.

When my daughter Charlotte was in the third grade, she was safely ensconced at a safe and nut-free school with happy social dynamics. She had been there since kindergarten and had even begun carrying her own EpiPen. We were feeling like we could take a breath and finally relax into a great routine. Then the unthinkable occurred. An impersonal, official letter arrived in the mail—without a word from anyone at the school—that briefly stated that at the end of the school year, the nut-free policy would be lifted and everyone could eat peanuts and tree nuts anywhere and everywhere, throughout the classrooms. This small school was in an old building without a cafeteria and equipped with an antiquated ventilation system—my severely allergic daughter would surely be exposed. The letter arrived well after the admissions timeline had ended for other schools. Its message was clear: Your medical condition is inconvenient, you're a nuisance, you impact what can and can't be put into kids' lunchboxes, so get out.

We were completely devastated. Indignant friends and supporters urged us to fight the school policy change with a lawyer, and one even stepped forward and offered to take our case for free. But we didn't have the heart. Why would we want our child to be in a place where she wasn't wanted? What kind of environment would this be for her, each day, if an administration forced by a legal system to "accommodate" grew hostile? No one wants to be someplace daily where he or she isn't welcome. Terrified, we began hustling to find another elementary school on extremely short notice. All the while, we politely grinned at the band of policy-making teachers and board parents we'd previously considered friends and supporters.

There is a silent aggression when facing other parents' feelings of inconvenience. They had to accommodate in-school snacks and needed to substitute sunflower butter for peanut butter in lunchboxes. Their backlash exercised control over us, as if punishing us for a disease we were just trying to manage. It was cruel. I even got Charlotte retested, hoping that maybe she would magically not be allergic anymore so that we could continue on in life without a major upheaval. But her numbers all came back sky high: still profoundly allergic. Things were looking very bleak for us.

Now there are much better food-labeling laws in place, and the overall awareness of food allergies is on the rise. But back then, when I broke the news to Charlotte, I struggled to answer her burning questions about why she couldn't stay at her school with her best friends. I myself didn't understand how this could happen: We'd moved houses to have decent proximity to her school, allergist, and the emergency room. We had tried to set her up for success the best we could.

Then, one afternoon, a clever and Internet-savvy friend found a ray of light: a small, very nice-looking elementary school with a welcoming and calm vibe. I called the school and made the inquiry: How could we keep a young child with a severe food allergy, surrounded by other young children, safe from exposure? The school was newly established, and to our utter surprise they were more than willing to put a nut-free safeguard in place to help our family. The kindness of the director and the thoughtfulness of the other parents were utterly refreshing. Cautiously, our broken hearts began to mend just a little. Charlotte spent a day at the school, and when I arrived to pick her up, my daughter and a sweet group of children all came tumbling out of the schoolroom together, breathlessly asking if Charlotte could please come back the following day. It all fell into place quickly, with a truly thoughtful group of teachers and parent body who are some of the warmest and loveliest people I've ever met. We'd found a safe, new school, a soft landing spot that would be completely nut-free.

The school was far away, actually very far away. It was well into another county and separated by the expansive Golden Gate

Bridge. And so, my nine-year-old daughter's medical condition led us to be separated each day by the ocean. Each day after school drop-off, I would head back home across the bridge.

Now, this particular bridge has a life of its own. There are stormy conditions so adverse that in the most extreme weather, the bridge closes to traffic. Lightning ferociously strikes it, and once it did so in broad daylight with us on it. Some people even take their own lives by jumping from it, and on my very first school drive I tragically witnessed how it is used as the second-most-common suicide site in the world. In our first month, an actual hunk of the bridge tore itself loose and crashed right into my windshield, leaving a bullet-hole-like circle in its wake. But the glass technician who came to repair it was utterly nonplussed as I held up the orange hunk of bridge; he had seen this repeatedly. During strong earthquakes, the bridge rocks and sways violently. And there's usually a fog warning on—which means driving into a looming, gray void that seems to have no beginning and no end. Sometimes the fog microclimate lasts for mere seconds, with blue light streaks suddenly showing through like a religious scene, and then just like that you are brilliantly awash in the happy Marin sunlight. Other times, a more stubborn, stickier, ominous fog envelopes you for miles, limiting visibility to the four feet in front of you. Fog spots dapple your vision as you feel along the bridge blindly.

I crossed this bridge four times daily: for a morning drop-off, then back home, and then an afternoon pickup, then mercifully home for the evening, my daughter safe and sound. I commuted back and forth like this for years, September through June, over and over. Which was okay because the Golden Gate Bridge is exceptionally expansive and beautiful. It was even declared a Wonder of the Modern World and is one of the most internationally recognized symbols of San Francisco and the United States.

The bridge is popular with pedestrians and bicyclists and, unlike most other bridges, was built with walkways. During the years I spent crossing the bridge, I witnessed nearly a dozen earnest wedding proposals, with one person down on a knee as the other squealed. I saw stumped tourists squinting into the fog, surprised to find themselves blanketed in freezing gray air, breathing and huffing out of their noses like dragons. And everyone had cameras poised to capture the magic—I even got into the habit of pulling over to take pictures of tourists for them. They came from all over the world, flocking to experience this site because, even in the freezing and fog and danger, it has a lot of magic.

All this time living in my beautiful Fog City, and I hadn't known what a power the bridge has. Both harrowing and stunning, it is just like living with food allergies: While traversing them both can indeed be dangerous, with masterful planning and design, it can also be the most beautiful journey you will ever take.

When Your Child Has Food Allergies

Part One

What You Need to Know

(1)

Food Allergy 101

FOOD ALLERGIES are common and becoming increasingly so. In 1980, 10 percent of the Western population suffered from allergies. Today, it is 30 percent. The Centers for Disease Control and Prevention reports that the prevalence of food allergies increased 18 percent in children between 1997 and 2007. According to the American College of Allergy, Asthma & Immunology, one in every thirteen children in the United States has a food allergy—which equals about two kids in every classroom.

Even though we don't have to face this alone, as parents of food-allergic children, we often feel that we do. Because even when we arm ourselves with facts and statistics, parents' perspectives are often marginalized in the diagnosis and treatment of food allergies. Many parents I work with feel relegated to the sidelines, even though they are the ones on the front lines. I think this feeling of alienation stems from the actual mystery of food allergy itself—with no cure, no known cause, and strict avoidance as the best treatment, no one quite knows what to do about it.

As food allergy parents, we look after our child's surviving and thriving but can sometimes feel as though schools, medical institutions, restaurants, and the hospitality industry find us to be polarizing and antagonizing. We essentially agree that our allergists are wonderful and well meaning, and we acknowledge that their work is delicate and absolutely involves the family as a whole. But they don't manage our child's allergy on a day-to-day basis like we do. When our child can't eat some foods and, in some rare cases, can't even breathe in the aromas without dire consequences, it's vital for us to make use of a blend of knowledge, lifestyle, and advocacy.

In this chapter, and all of the chapters that make up Part One of this book, I offer some of the knowledge that we can use to bridge any systemic or interpersonal gaps we encounter and ensure that we, as parents, can rise to this complex challenge.

KEY INFORMATION ON FOOD ALLERGIES

Here are some quick facts and statistics to have at your fingertips for caregivers, camps, group outings, and play dates:

Food allergies differ from other allergies because even a miniscule amount of the wrong food can be fatal. Dangerous trace amounts of the food, poorly processed and labeled foods, *cross-contaminated* utensils, or even particles carried on the unwashed hands and fingers of others pose a constant threat to children with food allergies.

There is no cure for a food allergy; only the strictest avoidance of the allergen can prevent an allergic reaction.

A food allergy develops when the body's immune system recognizes the food proteins as invaders and releases histamines and other chemicals to "attack."

Allergies to foods can cause *anaphylactic* reactions such as hives, nausea, closing of the breathing passages, a sudden drop in blood pressure, and even death.

More than eleven million Americans have food allergies of varying degrees of severity.

The number of children in the United States with peanut allergies has tripled over the past several decades.

Food allergies affect children and adults of all races and ethnicities and can develop at any age.

Children with food allergies must carry multiple doses of epinephrine in case of emergency. Epinephrine is the go-to, primary, best emergency treatment available to reduce the symptoms. Once epinephrine has been administered, the child must receive medical attention immediately—call 911!

The Difference Between an Allergy and a Sensitivity

It's important for parents and caregivers to know the difference between an allergic reaction and sensitivity to certain foods. Food sensitivity is also referred to as "food intolerance," which is a non-allergic hypersensitivity to a food that occurs when someone has difficulty digesting it. This can happen because elements of a certain food cannot be properly processed and absorbed by the digestive system. Most food sensitivities are generally less serious than an allergic reaction, and many are limited to digestive problems. Food allergies, on the other hand, trigger the immune system. For both food allergy and intolerance, currently there is no cure—so strict avoidance of the offending food is essential.

What Happens in an Allergic Response

An allergic reaction occurs when the body's immune system mistakenly attacks a food protein. The body overreacts, as if the food itself were harmful. In essence, the allergic immune system is miscalibrated, so it mistakenly targets proteins in certain foods as if they're harmful invaders of the body, like bacteria or viruses. The first time your child eats the food, his or her immune system makes an antibody called *immunoglobulin* (IgE), which attaches itself to cells that live in the nose, throat, lungs, skin, or gastrointestinal tract. Every time your child eats the offending food, these cells are activated to trigger a sudden release of chemicals, including histamine. This is when the symptoms surface. Severe allergic reactions can become cumulative, meaning that each time one is exposed to the offending food, the reaction becomes worse, as the histamines build up over time in the body. This can set the stage for the "perfect storm" of an allergic reaction, where even trace particles of the allergen, just a little leftover peanut butter on a spatula, can cause a full-blown and life-threatening reaction.

What Happens with Sensitivity

A food sensitivity, on the other hand, is manifested primarily by gastrointestinal symptoms such as a bloated feeling, flatulence, stomachache, nausea, or diarrhea. The most frequent and common sensitivities are to fructose (like sugar in fruit or fruit juice beverages and soft drinks) and lactose (a type of sugar found in dairy products). There is also wheat sensitivity to gluten, a protein found in wheat, barley, and rye. The science behind sensitivity is different than food allergy because food intolerances are caused by the partial or complete absence of activity of the enzymes responsible for breaking down or absorbing your food elements. There is a simple, noninvasive hydrogen breath test an allergist can easily administer to ascertain if a fructose or lactose sensitivity is the root cause of these described gut responses.

Some Clarity on Celiac Disease

Wheat allergy may sometimes be confused with celiac disease, but these conditions are very different—despite the fact that for both conditions, avoiding wheat and gluten is the primary treatment. A wheat allergy generates an allergy-causing antibody to proteins found in wheat. In people with celiac disease, gluten causes an abnormal immune system reaction in the small intestine, which damages it and interferes with absorption of food nutrients. When people with celiac disease eat foods or use products containing gluten, their immune system responds by damaging or destroying villi, finger-like protrusions lining the small intestine. Villi normally allow nutrients from food to be absorbed through the walls of the small intestine and into the bloodstream. Without healthy villi, you become malnourished, no matter how much food you consume. Typically, celiac disease presents with digestive symptoms, although in adults symptoms can vary greatly from person to person and present in unusual ways. There are other symptoms, including dermatitis herpetiformis, the skin manifestation of celiac disease. It is characterized by intensely itchy, chronic rashes that are usually found primarily on elbows, knees, back, buttocks, and back of neck. Discolored teeth can be a symptom of celiac disease, among other possible health issues. The symptom manifests as white, yellow, or brown spots on the front and back teeth (incisors and molars). Headaches can persist, as well as chronic tiredness.

Some patients develop symptoms of celiac disease early in life, while others feel healthy far into adulthood; my father, a medical doctor, developed celiac disease later in life. There are several blood tests available that screen for celiac disease antibodies, but the most common one is a tTG-IgA test. Celiac disease is a chronic autoimmune disease, which means that you can't outgrow it. The only current treatment for gluten sensitivity and celiac disease is avoiding all gluten-containing grains and sticking with a strict gluten-free diet.

As with food allergies, there is one striking similarity: The prevalence and awareness around celiac disease has made it easier to adapt and thrive with the condition since there are ample substitutions for foods available at supermarkets and at restaurants, and now that the diseases are well known, there is often empathy and assistance from the community at large to aid us.

Foods That Trigger Allergic Reactions

In 2004, the Food Allergen Labeling and Consumer Protection Act (FALCPA) identified eight major types of foods (which I call the "Big 8") that trigger allergic reactions and are required by law to be identified on labels when sold in the United States. You will learn to read labels carefully, as warnings such as "May contain milk" are voluntary and there are many names for each ingredient. If your child has an allergy to any of the following foods, I recommend that you scour the "Hidden Names" PDF downloads at www.kidswithfoodallergies.org. I offer some basic information here.

- **Milk:** This is the most common food that children are allergic to, at rates of 1 to 2 percent of children.
- **Eggs:** While it is the egg white that causes an allergic reaction, it is impossible to separate the yolk without leaving some trace of the egg white.
- **Finned fish:** This is often a lifelong allergy, and more than half of people allergic to one type of finned fish are also allergic to other types.
- **Crustacean shellfish:** Reactions to crustacea like shrimp, lobster, and crab tend to be particularly severe.
- **Peanuts:** This allergy is becoming ever more common. Between 1997 and 2008, the number of children allergic to peanuts in the United States tripled.
- **Tree nuts:** Tree nuts include walnut, almond, hazelnut, cashew, pistachio, and Brazil nuts, among others, and are totally different from peanuts (which are legumes).
- **Wheat:** This can be the most challenging food to avoid, since wheat is the most predominantly used grain in the United States.
- **Soy:** While soybeans in themselves are not a major part of this country's diet, they are extremely common in processed foods.

Early Preventative and Identification Measures

There is a vast number of contradictory theories about whether food allergies can be prevented. For example, for a while women were told to strictly avoid consuming nuts while pregnant, out of fear that it could cause food allergies in utero. Then the recommendation was reversed: Women were subsequently told it was better to consume plenty of the allergenic foods, in the hope of buttressing tiny immune systems as they developed. It's difficult to know which theories have validity, and as expecting mothers, we certainly don't want to perform any action that would *cause* food allergies!

However, the one thing allergy specialists seem to agree on is that breastfeeding infants has a protective effect to a point. A review of eighteen studies in the *Journal of the American Academy of Dermatology* found that allergy-prone children who were exclusively breastfed for three months were less likely to develop eczema—a rash often considered the first sign that a child is allergy prone—compared with those who were fed formula.

It's generally recommended that babies receive breastmilk for the first six months of their lives. It's least likely to trigger an allergic reaction, is easy to digest, and strengthens the infant's immune system. Especially recommended for the first four to six months, it may reduce early eczema, wheezing, and milk allergy.

For infants at risk for food allergy, if mom is unable to breastfeed, then hydrolyzed infant formulas are recommended over cow's milk and soy formulas since it's best to opt for a hypoallergenic formula, in which milk proteins are broken down so they won't provoke an immune response. There are also hypoallergenic soy-based formulas available if you find the milk is making your infant too colicky.

After your baby has reached the four- to six-month mark, with your pediatrician's recommendation, you can introduce solid foods carefully, one by one, starting with a food and sticking with it for a few days before moving on to the next one. New food can be introduced this way every few days, as appropriate for the infant's developmental readiness. This slow process gives parents a chance to identify and eliminate any food that appears to cause an allergic reaction.

Some doctors also recommend supplementing a child's diet with probiotics, intestinal bacteria that have a beneficial impact on health, to enrich intestinal flora. They've been used for decades to make yogurt. Probiotics have a proven effect on treating diarrhea, and studies are increasingly concluding that they have similar benefits for the immune system and allergies.

Possible Causes of Food Allergies

Allergies have been shown to be caused by family history, air pollution, processed foods, stress, and tobacco use. Currently, there are three major theories floating around about the causes of food allergies. The cause may be clear, or it may remain a complete mystery—which is okay since it won't affect how the allergy is treated.

Genetics and Heredity

Allergic diseases, such as asthma, allergic rhinitis (commonly known as hay fever), atopic dermatitis (also known as eczema), and food allergies tend to run in families. A child with one parent who has any kind of allergy, including environmental or seasonal allergies, has a 30 percent chance of becoming allergic. Having two allergic parents increases a child's risk to 60 percent. Just because you, your partner, or one of your children has an allergy doesn't mean that all of your kids will definitely get allergies. On the flip side, some kids develop allergies even if no family member is allergic.

Although the tendency to have allergies is inherited, how those allergies express themselves varies. They may occur in a very complex pattern because your child doesn't usually inherit your particular allergy, rather just the likelihood of having allergies. My daughter is a good example. She's highly allergic to peanuts and tree nuts while I'm highly allergic to fish. The only connection is that we're both highly allergic. Adding to this equation is that my parents are allergic, each to different Big 8 allergens, and so is my middle sibling (also to fish). A third sibling, the youngest, has no allergies at all—zero—which goes to show that you, your partner, or one of your children having allergies doesn't mean that all of your children will get them, too. Dr. Scott H. Sicherer, a leading national allergist, calculated the likelihood of peanut allergy in twins. His studies show that 7 percent of fraternal twins and two-thirds of identical twins share a peanut allergy, which affirms that genes and heredity do play a big role.

The Hygiene Hypothesis

Another major area of interest among researchers studying food allergies is the hygiene hypothesis. The popular hygiene hypothesis suggests that the overly sanitized state of our modern environment is upsetting the normal development of the immune system, leading to a possible overproduction of specific IgE antibodies. These IgE antibodies cause certain cells to release histamine, a protein that causes a variety of classic allergy symptoms. IgE antibodies are only found in mammals, and they are the bad guys that travel within the body to the cells, triggering them to release all of those histamines and chemicals, and causing the allergic reaction. The main premise of the hygiene hypothesis is that decreased exposure to germs and other disease-causing substances due to aspects of our modern Western lifestyles has decreased the human immune system's opportunity to develop standard immune responses. Because of this lack of opportunity, the immune system becomes prone to respond by reacting to otherwise harmless substances—in other words, by developing allergies.

Initially, scientists and researchers came up with the hygiene hypothesis. The original formulation of the hygiene hypothesis dates from the late 1980s and attempts to explain the disparity in patterns of allergic disease between North America and Western Europe and some other regions of the world. The hypothesis was put forth to explain why children raised on farms or with pets tend to have fewer allergies than children raised in cities and suburbs or without pets. Many experts firmly believe cleanliness is to blame for increasing allergies, according to Dr. Guy Delespesse, a professor at the Université de Montréal Faculty of Medicine. Our limited exposure to bacteria concerns Dr. Delespesse, who is also the director of the Laboratory for Allergy Research at the Centre Hospitalier de l'Université de Montréal. "There is an inverse relationship between the level of hygiene and the incidence of allergies and autoimmune diseases," says Dr. Delespesse in his paper "Why Are Allergies Increasing?" (University of Montreal, April 13, 2010). "The more sterile the environment a child lives in, the higher the risk he or she will develop allergies or an immune problem in their lifetime."

In 1980, 10 percent of the Western population suffered from allergies. Today, it is 30 percent. The mortality rate resulting from this affliction increased 28 percent between 1980 and 1994. In 2010, 1 out of 10 children was said to be asthmatic. "It's not just the prevalence but the gravity of the cases," says Dr. Delespesse. "Regions in which the sanitary conditions have remained stable have also maintained a constant level of allergies and inflammatory diseases."

Although hygiene does reduce our exposure to harmful bacteria, it also limits our exposure to beneficial microorganisms. As a result, the bacterial flora of our digestive system isn't as rich and diversified as it used to be. "Allergies and other autoimmune diseases such as Type 1 diabetes and multiple sclerosis are the result of our immune system turning against us," says Dr. Delespesse. Why does this happen? "The bacteria in our digestive system are essential to digestion and also serve to educate our immune system," adds Dr. Delespesse. "They teach it how to react to strange substances. This remains a key in the development of a child's immune system." Supplementing a child's diet with probiotics, as I discussed earlier, can help—as strange as it seems—their bodies to cope with environments that are so clean.

GMOs Under Suspicion

In 1996, genetically modified organisms, or GMOs, were introduced into our food supply. Genetically modified foods are produced from organisms that have had specific changes introduced into their DNA using methods of genetic engineering. Genes are inserted in seeds to make plants resistant to specific diseases or insects, to make plants easier to grow with less chemical weed killers, or to improve how plants ripen. According to a 2014 USDA Economic Research Service report, in 2000, 1 percent of the corn planted in the United States was genetically engineered; today, it's 90 percent, in addition to 93 percent of all soy. These crops show up as ingredients in an enormous number of foods and sodas under one name or another (high-fructose corn syrup or dextrose, for instance).

One early GMO horror story passed along to me that particularly resonated because of my severe allergy to seafood was that of the Frankenstein tomato, a strange hybrid of a tomato plant that was genetically engineered to resist frost. Scientists knew that the winter flounder fish had "antifreeze" in its blood to allow it to survive in extremely cold waters. They reasoned that putting antifreeze in plants would be incredibly useful since frost damage costs farmers hundreds of millions of dollars every year in lost crops or decreased productivity. The antifreeze in the fish is a protein called AFA3, which is coded to a gene. Fortunately, when this gene was tested in tomatoes, it didn't actually provide the much-anticipated frost resistance, so "fishy tomatoes" were never brought to market.

However, if they had been, it would have been an instructive example. If you cannot eat flounder without having an allergic reaction, you certainly could not eat these tomatoes—in ketchup, in marinara sauce at a pizza parlor, in soups in restaurants, in gravies served at holiday tables. The list could go on and on.

Every major scientific regulatory oversight body in the world, including both the National Academies of Science and the Food and Drug Administration in the United States, has concluded that genetically modified foods pose no harm. To date, there are no documented ill effects. Both regulatory and scientific agencies have developed international guidelines to address safety, with attention to nutrition, toxicity, and a variety of concerns in addition to allergies.

Still, a relationship between GMOs in the food supply and the increase in food allergies is a prevailing theory, despite reassurances, and the public remains curious and nervous regarding what the long-term impact of GMOs will be on our immunology. There have been multiple compelling case studies of GMOs and allergies. Most proteins are readily destroyed in our stomach and small intestine, broken down into their constituent amino acids and absorbed into our bloodstream, regardless of whether that protein comes from a cow or a tomato or a bacterium. Our

16

digestive systems and our immune systems are generally oblivious to their origin, but in this case, if we are what we eat, then are we what we eat . . . eats? Because food allergies can lead to anaphylaxis—and, worse, death—it's completely understandable that people are worried about the manipulation of our food supply.

It's impossible to claim that there's zero risk from using GMO technology in our food, but the possibility of risk alone is not a valid reason to avoid technology. We've embraced many technologies that have risks, from microwave ovens to cell phones, but there's more at stake here than quick meals or communication. To feed the billions of people on our planet without doing more irreparable harm to the environment, we must think about all options and all possibilities. This is the logic it's useful to consider to keep ourselves mindful and calm, not fearful of food and food allergies. A fear-based life is avoidable with in-depth information about the food our children eat, constant vigilance about what they eat, and rigorous education about the foods they can and cannot eat.

Possibility of Outgrowing Allergies

Can a child simply outgrow a food allergy? Can food allergies sometimes disappear as mysteriously as they arrived? Sometimes. Whether or not a food allergy can be outgrown depends largely on the type of food or foods to which your child is allergic. Many children allergic to milk, egg, wheat, or soy may outgrow their food allergy between three and sixteen years of age. The prognosis for other allergies, especially peanuts, tree nuts, and shellfish, is much different. They will rarely disappear when they are severe early in a child's life.

According to a study in the November 2005 *Journal of Allergy and Clinical Immunology*, only 9 percent of children with a tree nut allergy will ever outgrow this condition, and it's even less likely to be outgrown if a child is allergic to multiple types of tree nuts. Up to 20 percent of children with a peanut allergy have been shown to outgrow the allergy, and, again, if the child is allergic to multiple offenders, the allergy is less likely to be outgrown.

Researchers don't yet fully understand why some children grow out of their food allergies at a young age and why others never grow out of them. A 2013 study published in the *Annals of Allergy, Asthma and Clinical Immunology* revealed some new findings. First, the earlier a child had his of her first allergic reaction, the more likely that child was to potentially outgrow the food allergy. Second, boys were more likely than girls to outgrow their food allergy. The study also states that other factors that contributed to outgrowing an allergy included having a history of only mild to moderate reactions, being allergic to only one food, and having eczema as the only symptom. Conversely, children with severe symptoms, like trouble breathing, swelling, and anaphylaxis, as well as multiple food allergies, were less likely to achieve tolerance. It's tricky to know if children have outgrown their food allergies or if their tolerance to the allergen has increased.

Many families, including mine, reevaluate our child's food allergies annually with a visit to our allergist. This is the clearest way to tell if your child's numbers are going down. If you suspect that your child has been exposed on a few occasions to the allergen and there has been no visible symptoms of a reaction, it might seem tempting to feed just a bite of the allergen to see what happens, but this understandable eagerness could lead directly to anaphylaxis and tremendous respect for the serious potential consequences of food allergies. Instead, if you suspect your child may have outgrown food allergies (fingers crossed for you!)—for any reason—you should ask your allergist to perform formal testing before reintroducing and incorporating the foods into your family's meal planning.

2

Suspecting
Food
Is the Culprit

AS PARENTS, we know our children best. Having spent the first year with our little ones without speech and traditional conversation, parents have adapted to nonverbal cues and communication—our own perfect call and response with our infants. We are plugged directly into the vitality of our child's well-being. So it's no surprise that we can identify and understand when something is not quite right with our child's early eating habits and digestive health. Food is vital to help children grow up healthy and strong. With an ever-increasing number of kids developing allergies, parents become well aware that something as seemingly innocuous as a tuna fish sandwich, scrambled eggs, or a carton of chocolate milk can cause a chain reaction in which chemicals and histamines suddenly flood a child's body. And, naturally, whenever we watch that happen, it causes a surge of anxiety in us and we want to prevent it from ever happening again. But the struggle to avoid all traces of common food allergens can force allergic children to lead severely restricted lives—an effect that we would rather stave off by carefully attending to their environments.

One of the best ways to protect your children is to learn to read their symptoms. Whether mild or severe, you will need to be prepared to act in response. If you are at a stage in which you suspect food is causing your child to struggle, the following lists may help you know if you need to take that first step and schedule an appointment with a doctor or allergist.

Mild Early Warning Signs

Sometimes our children's allergies are all too apparent, but often—especially with our infants and toddlers—they are not. It's best to talk to a doctor as soon as possible about any of these symptoms:

- Eczema
- Hives, rashes, or itching
- Diarrhea that is frequent
- Swelling that is mild and does not affect breathing or blood pressure
- Vomiting as a response to ingesting formula or food
- Wheezing

When to Call an Ambulance

It's essential to watch out for these severe and sudden symptoms and to teach your child to speak up when he or she is not feeling well—because a food allergy can be potentially fatal. If any of these reactions manifest, immediately call an ambulance:

- Dramatic drop in blood pressure
- Loss of consciousness
- Trouble breathing or inability to breathe
- Vomiting violently and repeatedly

General Symptoms of Food Allergies

Following are the signs and symptoms that are often caused by food allergies. If any of these are familiar to you, immediately begin recording each time it shows up in your child and note what he or she last ate. This will help you communicate your concerns to a doctor or allergist.

- Behavior problems
- Chronic cough
- Circles under eyes that are dark and purplish
- Colds that are frequent
- Coughing at night, with a stuffy nose in the morning
- Diarrhea, abdominal pain, and bloating
- Ear infections that happen frequently
- Fatigue
- Headaches
- Intestinal gas after eating that is severe
- Itchiness or swelling in the mouth, face, lips, or throat
- Runny nose with clear secretions
- Skin rashes, such as eczema or hives, that are chronic or frequent
- Sneezing
- Watery eyes
- Wheezing breath

Symptoms of Anaphylaxis

Anaphylaxis is a severe, life-threatening allergic reaction that can develop in seconds. Basically, a child's body gets so flooded by chemicals in response to an allergen that it goes into shock. This is categorized as a medical emergency, so if you suspect this is occurring, don't think: Call an ambulance. The following is a list of signs and symptoms often caused by anaphylaxis:

- Bluish (cyanotic) lips and mouth area
- Change of voice
- Coughing
- Diarrhea
- Difficulty breathing, shortness of breath
- Difficulty swallowing
- Dizziness, change in mental status
- Fainting or loss of consciousness
- Flushed, pale skin
- Itching of any body part
- Itchy, scratchy lips, tongue, mouth, or throat
- Red, watery eyes
- Runny nose
- Sense of doom
- Stomach cramps
- Swelling of any body part
- Throat tightness or closing
- Vomiting
- Wheezing

Symptoms of Eosinophilic Esophagitis

Eosinophilic esophagitis (EE) is an allergic response that has only recently been recognized and is increasingly found in food-allergic children. It is an inflammatory reaction of the esophagus, the muscular tube that carries food from the throat to the stomach. Eosinophils are a type of white blood cell that are not normally found in the esophagus, so high levels of them indicate an allergic response.

The presence of eosinophils in the esophagus causes inflammation in the gastrointestinal tract, which makes digestion very painful. Its symptoms mimic gastroesophageal reflux disease (GERD). Here are some of the symptoms associated with EE.

- Abdominal pain
- Chest pain
- Choking
- Cramping
- Diarrhea
- Difficulty swallowing
- Failure to thrive
- Nausea
- Reflux not relieved by standard antireflux therapy
- Vomiting
- Weight loss

Studies have revealed that EE symptoms do not improve with aggressive acid blockage therapy used to treat GERD. They do improve with an elimination diet or corticosteroid treatment. The skin prick test and patch testing (discussed in chapter 3) can help identify which foods may contribute to this disease. The foods most commonly associated with EE are cow's milk, soy, egg, and wheat. Airborne allergens may also contribute to a reaction. Many children with this disorder have more than one allergy problem.

How I Discovered My Daughter's Allergy

My own standard twenty-week ultrasound did not show or predicate that my child would be born with food allergies. There was no birthmark or visual deficiency that gave this away on the day of her birth. I was just thrilled that she had all her fingers and toes. I was—if you will forgive the word—"lucky" that I have severe, in fact, anaphylactic, food allergies myself, so at least I had a logical understanding that the possibility existed that my child, carrying my DNA, could also suffer from my hereditary medical condition.

The discovery was still painful, traumatic, scary, and disappointing—even with the logical DNA piece I well understood. At age three, a terrifying lone bite of a friend's peanut butter sandwich sent us racing to the emergency room, and nothing was ever the same again. Instantly, my daughter began projectile vomiting and her face began to balloon and swell. There literally wasn't even time to call for an ambulance as I witnessed the rapid onset of her allergic reaction. I grabbed her, all but tossed her into her car seat, and zoomed us to the emergency room.

I felt powerless as I watched a million life opportunities wash away in my mind's eye in that instant. It seemed so unfair to have to mourn a life lived free of this life-threatening medical condition before it had even really begun. I succumbed to the grief only a parent could know: Would my daughter survive her food allergies? Could she endure it? Could I? The world crushed down around me, so unfair, cruel, even.

Then I plastered on my smile, put my little one in her shiny new Maclaren stroller, and gathered up my diaper bag, and off we headed to the playground—because what else can you do? Life moves on, and I wanted her to enjoy the blissful moments of being young, playing, developing basic skills, and just existing. Always tactile and sensitive, she dug her new hands into the sand over and over, just feeling the sensation. I looked up at the clouds and beyond, helpless and hopeful at the same time, cursing and thanking the cosmos.

And, spoiler alert: Yes, of course we did find our way, with incredible support and input from my daughter's pediatrician, whose own father became our beloved family allergist. Piece by piece, brick by brick, we systematically and vigilantly forged our own specific allergy action plan, which worked and still works for us.

From the birthing suite all the way onward to college, your food-allergic child's life path can bloom beautifully despite the harrowing beginning.

3

Food
Allergy Diagnosis
Options

THERE ARE SEVERAL COMPLAINTS and signs your children may provide that can serve as clues about what foods they are allergic to. When my daughter was young, she once complained that a bite of lasagna caused an alarming "poking" and sharp sensation in her mouth; she could even point to the exact spot. It was, in fact, her nut allergy flaring up due to cross-contaminated restaurant lasagna. Other times, children will complain endlessly about eating a certain food, often loudly protesting and saying repeatedly that they don't like it. They might say that it feels weird on their tongues or in their throats, that it's hard to swallow, or that it's just plain "yuck." Their aversion seems heightened and not normal—and it often persists. All of these are signs you can use when trying to identify a food allergy. This chapter offers an overview of the methods that are helpful to diagnose the problem.

Medical History

Your child's medical history is of tremendous value when diagnosing a food allergy. During your first visit, the doctor or allergist will most likely ask you a series of probing questions to determine whether your suspicions are well founded. You can prepare for the doctor's review by carefully documenting your answers to these questions:

- At what age did your child's suspected food allergy begin?
- What were the specific symptoms?
- Did the child's reaction occur soon after eating the suspect food?
- Does a reaction always occur when he or she eats that food?
- Had he or she ever previously tolerated that food?
- How much was consumed before there was any kind of reaction?
- Did anyone else who ate the same food get sick with similar or different symptoms?
- How was the food prepared? Was it homemade or store bought?
- What food(s) do you suspect your child is allergic to?

Your answers to these questions, along with a food allergy diary and allergy log, will be instrumental in providing your allergist with a well-rounded recent history. A parent's instinct and observations, combined with a child's personal feedback, are the most important and useful diagnostic tools to identify any consistent patterns in allergic reactions.

Food Diary and Allergy Log

Be prepared for your doctor to ask you to keep a food diary of what your child eats and his or her reactions to it. It might even be a good idea to arrive in the doctor's office with the diary in hand. A good food diary will have room to record each meal, every day of the week, and to rate the reaction on a scale of 1 to 10, whether the effect is symptoms, digestion, energy, or mood. You can find many diaries online by searching for "food allergy diary template." Just print out many copies of the one you like and you're good to go.

Another great tool to use alongside the food diary is an allergy log, which corresponds the leading allergen sources directly with any symptoms your child may experience as a result of exposure. These can also be found with a simple online search.

Yes, keeping track of everything your child eats is labor intensive for a while, but it will help your doctor to know which tests to order.

Elimination Diet

An elimination diet relies on trial and error to identify specific allergies and intolerances. Basically, different foods and possible allergens are removed from the child's environment until symptoms disappear. Then, one by one, the substances are reintroduced back into the child's menu until one triggers a reaction. Typically, if symptoms resolve after the removal of a food from the diet, then the food is reintroduced (in a small dose) to see whether the symptoms reappear. This sort of challenge-dechallenge-rechallenge approach is particularly useful in cases with intermittent or vague allergic symptoms.

Skin Tests

Realistically, there's no such thing as a completely stress-free, unobtrusive, painless allergy test. Skin tests involve pricks with tiny needles, and they do not go very deep. But this patch skin test is still uncomfortable, especially for young children. While it is relatively painless, that's small comfort for a little one when it's time for the test.

The skin test determines a reaction to particular foods by placing a diluted, tiny extract of the suspected food on the skin of a child's back. This portion of the skin is then pricked with a needle to allow a tiny amount of the food extract beneath the skin surface. Then the area is observed for swelling or redness, called a *wheal*, which has the appearance and the feel of a mosquito bite. Its appearance signifies a local allergic reaction to the allergen. If, for example, your child is allergic to egg protein but not to wheat, then only the egg allergen will cause a little swelling or itching. The spot where the wheat allergen was applied will remain normal.

In some highly allergic people—especially if they have had anaphylactic reactions—skin tests should not be done because they could provoke another dangerous reaction. Skin tests also cannot be done on children with extensive eczema, as it could make things even worse.

The good news is that with skin tests you don't have to wait long to find out what is triggering allergies. Reactions occur within about twenty minutes and many begin to go away within thirty minutes. Generally there won't be any other symptoms besides the small bumps where the tests are positive. A positive test signifies that the child has the immunoglobulin E (IgE) antibody specific to the food being tested. You can keep Benadryl and a topical antihistamine or hydrocortisone ointment on hand, but many allergists suggest that these should only be administered after the test is completed so that the result is clear. Only once did I have an unusual and unexpectedly severe reaction to a skin test for grass pollen—as an adult, surprisingly—when my little wheal swelled up almost to a regulation baseball size. I was forced to take the oral antihistamine Benadryl for two days straight. But rest assured, that's not common for a patch skin prick test.

Skin tests are rapid, simple, and relatively safe. But a positive reaction to this test alone isn't definitive enough to confirm a food allergy because a child can have a positive skin test to a food allergen without experiencing allergic reactions to that food. A doctor typically diagnoses it as a food allergy only when the patient has a positive skin test to a specific allergen and the child's history suggests an allergic reaction to the same food.

Blood Tests

A more comprehensive way to measure an immune system response to particular foods is by checking the amount of IgE antibodies in your child's bloodstream. For this test, a small blood sample is taken either in your doctor's office or directly at a medical laboratory where different foods can be tested. Your child may need to avoid taking certain medicines like antihistamines one to several days before the test because they might affect the test result. It's a good idea to make sure the pediatrician or allergist knows about any medicines, herbs, or supplements that your child takes when scheduling the test.

Regular testing is important. My daughter and I test annually to understand the baseline numbers and read them ourselves to ensure that we're not dealing with false positive results. As with positive skin tests, positive blood tests confirm the diagnosis of a specific food allergy only when the tests are compatible with the clinical history. In our cases, they are.

Since the blood test is pretty traumatic for younger children, we prefer to have ours performed at a small, private lab we found by researching online. There are fewer folks there, and that helps a child who's already feeling self-conscious and trying to work up the nerve to give blood for the test. Preparing your child at home and during the car ride is key. Take it from me, promising "it won't hurt" or "it only takes a second" isn't very effective or even remotely truthful. Instead, a calm but rational explanation rooted in truth works best: "This is the best way to find out if you're still allergic. I really need to know; I want to know. Don't you want to know?" Food-allergic children have to be so much more self-governing and careful than other kids, and even though they're young, they know the stakes and understand the limitations of their medical condition.

Not much is as daunting as taking your child into a cold, sterile office and handing over the paperwork for the radioallergosorbent (RAST) allergy blood test. Plain and simple, blood must be drawn from your child's arm. You can try quietly asking, in advance, for your lab technician to use a butterfly needle at the injection site, which is much smaller than even the regular gauge used on children. It's less scary, it doesn't hurt nearly as much, and even the name sounds more pleasant to little ears.

You could have some distractions at the ready for the big moment; this time-tested parental trick can help reduce the pain. Even the slightest diversions can eliminate problems. My treasure chest of successful distractions includes playing with a new toy, pointing out a picture on the wall, reciting ABCs, telling your child something funny, or even blowing bubbles. Try your best to keep smiling through the blood draw, even though it's difficult, because many children will take their cues directly from their parent or caregiver in a time of crisis. It's unrealistic to imagine the two of you will be grinning through this lab appointment, but if you can provide even just that little bit more levity, the time will pass more quickly, with less trauma, for the little patient. Some older children feel better hugging their parent, chest to chest, when blood is drawn. If your doctor believes it's appropriate, allowing older kids to choose the right or left arm themselves may provide them with a sense of some control over the phlebotomy process.

In the end, a minor bribe might not feel like a parenting crime during such a necessary—yet traumatic—situation as bloodwork on a very little, uncertain, and frightened child. A trip for ice cream (as long as you do not suspect your child is allergic to milk or egg) or to a favorite toy store or destination immediately afterward could help a young person soldier through with a tangible goal and a reward to focus on.

4

Treatments
for
Food Allergies

YOU MAY HEAR a lot about ongoing studies that are seeking new treatment options for food allergies. This is because there are not very many tried-and-true treatments. We know what will stop an allergic reaction, but we have no proven way to prevent it and no way to overcome the allergy completely. Here is an overview of what we know—and don't know—about managing food allergy symptoms.

Medical ID Bracelets Can Be Fun

Alert others to your child's allergies with a medical ID alert bracelet because they can let others know what is happening even if your child can't. You can personalize a bracelet so that it details your child's specific allergies and also expresses the child's own individual and fun tastes. Kid-friendly options are available from companies such as AllerMates and Allerbling, and your child can choose his or her own favorite style and design. All of these small steps in advance can expedite a diagnosis and solution at the ER.

Epinephrine Is Your Go-To Solution

Once a severe allergic reaction starts, epinephrine is the first line of defense. It's a synthetic adrenaline that can reverse the severe symptoms of an allergic reaction in seconds. Loaded into an auto-injectable device, one shot can stop an allergic reaction in its tracks, and because of this, it's considered the first and best solution to combat food allergies once they have been triggered.

Unlike antihistamine tablets and syrups like Benadryl, which can be only vaguely useful, epinephrine is available by a prescription only. For me and millions of others, the most trusted, go-to solution for epinephrine is the EpiPen auto-injector. Other devices have come and gone from the pharmaceutical marketplace, and several are being tested. One that functioned with a long-lasting battery and talked users through the process has been recalled and removed from the marketplace.

The EpiPen administers a dose of epinephrine when injected into a person's thigh during an allergic reaction. Injecting epinephrine directly into the thigh delivers the medicine throughout the body faster than taking an oral dose of antihistamine, which would have to be digested before entering the bloodstream. The epinephrine then raises dangerously low blood pressure by tightening the blood vessels. Epinephrine in the blood eases breathing by helping the lung muscles relax and reduces swelling in the throat and face. Then the heart rate increases as blood pressure rises, delivering the epinephrine faster to the whole body.

History of the EpiPen

The EpiPen was originally derived from the ComboPen, a military product developed to treat exposure to nerve agents in the 1960s. The inventor, Sheldon Kaplan, was a former NASA engineer. Kaplan modified the ComboPen to be a delivery device for epinephrine, thus creating the EpiPen. The device contains a spring-loaded needle that exits the tip of the pen, penetrating the recipient's skin and delivering the medication via an intramuscular injection. Kaplan patented the EpiPen in 1977, but it wasn't until the 1980s that the EpiPen was made available to the public for use with a prescription.

Obtaining a Prescription

Once you have a food allergy diagnosis, you will most likely receive a prescription for epinephrine auto-injectors, typically in two-packs. Your allergist will determine whether your child should start with the junior-strength auto-injector or a full-strength auto-injector based on his or her weight. Prescription auto-injectors can be pricey, depending on your state. But they are worth it, as auto-injectors are always the best line of defense for food allergies and anaphylaxis. Check with your health insurance carrier. You can also surf the Internet and look at pharmaceutical websites because there are periodically coupons, offers, and specials available to help defray the cost. Sometimes there are even coupons that offer free copays.

How to Use an EpiPen

The EpiPen is a patented device that administers a dose of epinephrine when injected into the user's thigh following an allergic reaction. There are three simple steps for using an EpiPen.

1. Remove the blue safety cap so the device can deploy, and depress the auto-injector until you hear a distinct clicking sound.
2. Once you hear the click, hold the EpiPen in place for ten seconds to allow the epinephrine to fully empty from the needle.
3. Then massage the site to help speed the drug into the bloodstream.

Don't Relax—Call an Ambulance

Once the symptoms of a severe allergic reaction ease, you must go to an emergency room for continued treatment and evaluation by a medical professional. There can be a secondary reaction—known as a biphasic reaction—that occurs once the EpiPen injection wears off. This means the allergic person has a second reaction that occurs two to six hours after the first reaction, often when the first wave of symptoms is under control. This reaction can be even more symptomatic and dangerous than the first. Therefore, a period of monitoring in a medical setting, such as the nearest emergency room, for at least six hours is the safest course of action after a severe allergic reaction.

Current practical medical advice: Delayed use of epinephrine during an anaphylactic allergic reaction has been associated with death, so when in doubt, administer the epinephrine and call 911 because the risks associated with not using the pen outweigh any side effects of epinephrine.

Practice Using the Auto-Injector

Practice makes perfect. Each family member, and especially the allergic child himself or herself, can be prepared to respond in an emergency. Your little one can be taught quite early how to self-administer these lifesaving meds into his or her outer thigh, just in case. A standard EpiPen brand epinephrine auto-injector two-pack includes a "trainer," which is designed to perfectly replicate the device but contains no medicine and no needle. Unlike the real pen, where a needle comes out once the syringe tip is pushed against a person's leg, it can be used again and again and no one is ever injected. The trainer and the real pen are visually different, so everyone in the family who spends time with your child can safely practice how to deploy the EpiPen.

Because the trainer is for practice only, be sure to keep it separate from your child's rescue medication. In an emergency, seconds count, and the trainer can't dispense the lifesaving medication.

Competition Heating Up for Epinephrine Solutions

While the EpiPen currently dominates the market share ever since a compact battery-operated device named Auvi-Q was voluntarily recalled in late 2015; the owners of their voice-guided auto-injector announced in October 2016 that the device will be back on the market in 2017. This has been welcome news for food allergy families amid a controversy which began in July 2016 over the Mylan EpiPen price hike when it surfaced that the list price for their epinephrine auto-injectors had suddenly hit $600 or as high as $1,000 for families with high health plan policyholder deductions. In response, Mylan will also offer a $300 list price generic version of their EpiPen two-pack with updated packaging and so there is relief—and options—in sight.

Advice for Carrying an Epinephrine Auto-Injector

Epinephrine is only administered to control symptoms after a reaction occurs, and it's essential to carry your auto-injector of epinephrine with you at all times. It's an even better idea to carry two in the extremely rare case that one malfunctions or is not sufficient to reduce the symptoms of anaphylaxis until appropriate medical treatment is available. Once your child enters the second grade, you should encourage him or her to carry a rescue medicine bag containing the medications.

You must not ever store your child's auto-injectors in a car glove box: Epinephrine should not be subjected to extreme heat or extreme cold. There are many options for carrying cases that are available everywhere, from the charming Etsy craft website to your local pharmacy. It's best to get used to carrying the medication with you, on your person, at all times when you leave the house, especially when your child is newly diagnosed and you are adjusting to several lifestyle changes at once.

The Emergency Room Is the Safest Place to Be After a Reaction

Once the symptoms of a severe allergic reaction ease, you must still go to an emergency room for continued treatment and evaluation by a medical professional. After using epinephrine, even if the symptoms of a severe allergic reaction ease, you should further seek emergency medical attention by calling 911 immediately and informing dispatchers that you have just used epinephrine for a suspected food-induced anaphylactic reaction.

An ambulance can provide more than just a speedy trip to the emergency room: The paramedics or emergency medical technicians on board can provide medication and IV fluids on the way. Most significantly, and with every second counting, paramedics can also inform the emergency room of your condition before you arrive. At the emergency room, they'll administer continued treatment and evaluation in a safe place for symptom observation.

Emergency room staff knows how difficult it can be for family members to remain calm in the face of an emergency, but do your best to remain laser focused on the task at hand: providing support and comfort to your child while at the hospital. You do not ever need to leave your child completely alone in a hospital, and someone should always stay with your child as emergency room staff decide on the treatment plan. Some hospitals might limit this to one person if the emergency room is very crowded or if a procedure needs to be performed, but the rest of the gang can still be in the waiting room and can ask when to return and come back in.

Emergency Room Visits on the Rise

The rate of emergency room visits for food allergies and anaphylaxis has skyrocketed and doubled from 2005 to 2014. A Mayo Clinic study determined this information using a nationwide administrative claims database: the highest increase noted was observed in kids aged 5–17. In this age bracket, the anaphylaxis increased by 196 percent, and reactions to foods went up 285 percent. The study was unable to determine if these increases are attributed to a better understanding of food allergies and anaphylaxis, or more accurate hospital coding systems, but all agree it points towards a need for greater overall food allergy awareness and clearer and swifter diagnoses in order to protect this group.

Epinephrine Is—Always—Your First and Best Line of Defense

The only reason I mention antihistamines, like Benadryl, is that they are good to carry in an emergency bag. But they should never be solely relied on with anaphylaxis. While useful for allergic rhinitis, hay fever, or a mild allergic reaction, antihistamines as a standalone are not a lifesaving solution for a severe anaphylactic allergic reaction. Drill this message into your family's food allergy noggins: *When in doubt, use the EpiPen.* Generally, antihistamines are secondary to assist. So unless specifically instructed by your allergist, if there has been ingestion of your allergen, always use epinephrine at the first sign of a reaction—hopefully before things start to spiral out of control. The current food allergy wisdom is that with a severe and potentially life-threatening allergic reaction, the dangers involved outweigh mistakenly using the epinephrine auto-injector and its potential side effects.

Relaxation Therapies Can Ease Symptoms

Stress is our body's response to situations, inside and out, that interfere with the normal balance in our lives. Virtually all of our body's systems—digestive, cardiovascular, immune, and nervous—make adjustments in response to stress. So when we are under intense stress, our bodies actually release hormones and other chemicals, including histamine, which is the powerful chemical that causes allergy symptoms.

Stress can make an allergic reaction far worse by increasing the histamine flooding a child's bloodstream. And chronic stress that persists for weeks or even months produces cortisol, the body's main stress-induced hormone. When cortisol becomes elevated and remains so for a significant length of time, it affects the cells that comprise our immune system, causing a chain reaction: The immune system can't keep infections or diseases at bay as it normally does. Viruses or bacteria proliferate to the point where they can infect many cells, leading to increased chance of illness and weakness.

Research shows that stress can aggravate allergic reactions, even a full day after an anxiety-producing event. That might be because as stress hormones rise in your body, so do levels of *cytokines*—proteins we produce as part of the allergic response. Cytokines are any of a number of substances secreted by specific cells in the immune system, which carry signals locally between cells and thus have an effect on other cells. Researchers at Ohio State University found that not only did allergy attacks become stronger when a person was going through significant anxiety and stress, but they also lasted longer, often moving on to a second or third day after the initial attack was over. Those suffering from allergies likely developed anxiety separately from their allergies, but their anxiety still affected their allergic reactions, creating a vicious cycle.

The Complicated Relationship Between Allergies and Stress

But can stress *cause* allergy symptoms? Respected scientists have revealed groundbreaking evidence on the effect of stress on overall immune function. A study by Dr. Gailen D. Marshall, professor of medicine and pediatrics at the University of Mississippi, was performed on forty-five medical students taking final exams to see if stress negatively affected their resistance to disease. The students were studied three to four weeks prior to exams and then again during exams to see how they responded to a hepatitis vaccine. Compared to students who received the vaccine under relaxed conditions, the stressed students showed much weaker immune system responses to the vaccine. It makes sense that stress affects immune response.

But how about allergies? The relationship between allergies and stress is complicated. Each person's body reacts differently, both to allergies and to stress, so it's difficult for researchers to pinpoint the cause and effect without further clinical study. For researchers to understand the relationship, they would have to test children regularly on stress and allergy measurement scales from a young age over the course of years. Nevertheless, researchers have come up with several theories on the relationship:

- Certain allergies cause changes to the brain and the body, which internally cause stress.
- Living with allergies causes stress and discomfort, which may cause people to develop anxiety.
- Allergies do not cause anxiety, but they make anxiety worse.
- Allergies have no effect on anxiety, but anxiety makes allergies worse.
- Allergies and anxiety are independent of each other, but they may have some common conditions between them that cause changes in immune system health.

Researchers have found that any one of these could potentially be true and that it is even more likely that all of them are true—differently for different people. This much is already clear: Allergy symptoms are an example of an overreaction by the immune system to otherwise harmless substances, and recurring stress can exacerbate an allergy.

Whether allergies in and of themselves can physiologically be the root cause of physical stress and anxiety is still being studied. What some theorize is more likely: the constituent physical and mental demands of living with allergies place additional stress on our bodies. All chronic stress has the potential to contribute to anxiety, and it also hurts quality of life, which in turn affects anxiety and stress levels. In this sense, allergies are causing anxiety, but the specific reactions as a result of allergies are not the direct cause.

The most likely scenario is that the two are independent but affect each other. Allergy attacks likely make anxiety worse because they cause a poorer quality of life and physical symptoms that may contribute to further anxiety. Anxiety makes allergies worse by altering the immune system and releasing more allergy-causing hormones. Together, they become a cyclical problem that may not stop without some intentional de-stressing techniques. You may feel added stress when some family and friends (or even annoying total strangers) find it hard to believe that, with a new diagnosis, one bite or less of an allergen really can lead to an extreme allergic reaction or even loss of life.

Counseling Can Help Everyone

If your child's allergy is contributing to his or her experience of anxiety, there is plenty you can do to control it. Anxiety is an emotional reaction despite having a physical cause, so learning to combat anxious thought processes can aid a high quality of life. Counseling is helpful for children to learn ways to relate to very real risks.

Your own firm approach is completely appropriate, and when all else fails, you have to put politeness aside and be assertive about making your child's food allergy needs crystal clear. Remember, your child's life can be endangered by even the most well-meaning person who does not understand the importance of strict avoidance of allergenic foods and who thinks just a lick or a small taste is insignificant and okay. Your diligence about your child's environment can help him or her relax within it. But if you are on red alert all the time, your own health will suffer, so counseling can help you manage stress, too.

If you and your family members are experiencing feelings of depression or isolation, don't hesitate to seek support or counseling. Because, the deal is, we can't always flex our families to appear like others who enjoy a lifestyle that doesn't involve the daily challenge of life-threatening food allergies. People's lack of understanding about food allergies, a lot of times, is just ignorance. What you can do is create a lifestyle for you and your family that is both fun and as "normal" and healthy as possible. Accept the fact that you can no longer have such a carefree approach to your child's foods, and do your best to maintain a positive attitude as we wait for a cure.

Oral Immunotherapy Within a Clinical Setting

On the pioneering edge of food allergy research are clinical studies for oral immunotherapy (OIT). This is a treatment where your child ingests small amounts of the allergen. While this might seem contraindicatory—the opposite of the strict avoidance that's generally advocated—it's not as terrifying as it might sound. This is because the amount initially ingested in these studies is merely particles; in fact, more like a particle of a particle—and only in a supervised, medical setting as an organized part of a clinical trial performed at a hospital, with qualified doctors and a team present.

Children start these clinical studies by swallowing microscopic specks of their allergen on a daily basis at the medical facility, with nurses standing by and epinephrine close at hand. If patients can manage the infinitesimal amounts without suffering an allergic reaction, the team progresses to a tiny bit larger daily dose, then a bit bigger again, and on it goes until it reaches the level that causes an allergic response. This is how a baseline is determined for these tests, and once the allergic reaction level is established, the trained medical team begins to work with its little patients to establish "desensitization" toward the allergenic food. As the process evolves, to keep up the desensitization, a "maintenance dose" of the allergen (typically four grams) must be eaten every day at home in the years that follow. For example, if a child allergic to peanuts has been desensitized to six whole peanuts, he or she must continue to eat the same quantity daily and never, ever skip a day.

The Theory Behind It

The thesis behind OIT involves slowly desensitizing the immune systems of highly allergic children by feeding them gradually increasing amounts of whatever they're allergic to, with the goal of slowly boosting their ability to tolerate those allergenic foods. While not a cure, this program in a clinical setting enables some food-allergic children to consume reasonably small amounts of foods they were previously allergic to and not experience an allergic reaction. This is useful in case of an accidental ingestion or a cross-contamination or cross-contact.

The problem is that people hear partial information about such studies and—understandably—imagine that now there is a food allergy cure. Grandparents, an excited aunt, well-meaning dear friends enthusiastically call families and announce: Have you heard the great news? All you have to do is feed your child the almonds, a little at a time, and he or she will build up a natural immunity! However, the strict reality is that you cannot try this type of food challenge at home yourselves because there is a pharmaceutical component that is involved in the clinical trials. A suppressing drug is regularly administered to all of the children at the medical facility as an integral part of the trial. This is to increase the likelihood that the child will have either no or only a small allergic reaction to the allergen particles.

Additional Medication

One world-renowned, global leader in medical care and OIT research is Stanford Medical Center, which is striving to develop new therapies for food-allergic disorders. Their studies include a wide range of patients who represent a diverse group of ethnicities and socioeconomic backgrounds. Every Stanford clinical test subject in the OIT study is given the medication XOLAIR, and only then are the allergic particles administered. XOLAIR is prescribed for severe allergic asthma. This particular medication also reduces sensitivity to inhaled or ingested allergens. It has been on the market for years and has been used in various clinical trials for more than fifteen years. While pricey, it is neither new nor experimental, is well established, and is very reputable. So, dosing a child with this drug in a safe medical setting prior to even the smallest nibble of their allergen provides solid protection. Like all drugs, however, this prescribed medicine can cause adverse side effects depending on the individual—which is to be expected.

It Might Help, It Might Not

Even with all of the research on various food allergies and OIT, some young children enrolled in these studies continue, despite the suppressing medication, to have serious and scary allergic reactions during and even after they have completed the trial. Their families have to deeply commit to the study and stay engaged for two full years until the desensitization process is completed under the watchful eye of the experts. After that time, the children are able to resume their normal lives, except they must continue to consume the maximum allotment of the allergen they ate while in the study. They can't taper off or eliminate it completely from their diets. It's too soon to call these studies "cures" because long-term tolerance has not yet been adequately assessed.

Not surprisingly, this is a debated approach with many pros and cons and very strong opinions on both sides. Sometimes doctors associated with a series of studies this groundbreaking are considered "outlaws" and "cowboys" or, inversely, "allergy busters" and "saviors." Understandably, when a family feels too inhibited by a food allergy to function effectively and perform regularly in day-to-day life, the risk of trying something—anything—new might seem, while perhaps risky, like the only stone left unturned. Having met some of the families participating in these studies, it's easy to understand their frustration and impatience with more conventional therapies. But my severely allergic family and I have opted not to try this course of action.

OIT is a step forward during this tremendously dynamic time for food allergy awareness. It's understandable that parents often have high hopes of halting this accelerating public health issue and unlocking a complex riddle with seemingly no answer. After all, if our society doesn't attempt to take risks and to conquer new hurdles, even with radical measures, how can we find the food allergy solution and a lifesaving cure?

Traditional Chinese Medicine

Some new clinical trials are under way in the United States for a formula called food allergy herbal formula 2 (FAHF-2). FAHF-2 is based on a long-used traditional Chinese medicine formula for parasite infection. In early scientific testing, which blends a combination of both Eastern and Western medicinal practices, it has been found to completely block anaphylaxis in mouse models. In time and with more research, this could provide another avenue for a food allergy solution. In 2016, Mount Sinai Hospital in New York opened the Center for Chinese Herbal Therapy, which focuses on researching the use of these herbal medicines, and even acupuncture, in specific allergic disorders. They have even established a Botanical Chemistry Lab with advanced equipment and technology to fully understand the combination of herbs to develop possible future food allergy medications.

Strict Avoidance

An allergic reaction to food can affect the skin; the gastrointestinal tract; the respiratory tract; and, in the most serious cases, the cardiovascular system. There are promising new clinical trials to fight food allergies, but to date no medication can be taken to prevent food allergies. The only viable method for managing food allergies so far is avoiding allergens and treating emergencies when they occur.

Integrating this approach into your lifestyle and environment is essential to making it work. And that is what the rest of this book is about.

Part Two

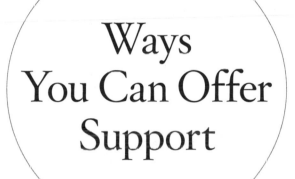

Ways
You Can Offer
Support

5

Talking to
Your Child at Any Age
About Staying Safe

AN ALLERGIC REACTION can be a scary thing. Younger children may not be able to fully understand their allergies, let alone explain them to other children or adults. Whether it's a mild reaction or a more severe one, children will likely remember the discomfort and irritation they felt during the response. For a child, the fear of having another reaction can be paralyzing. It's important to help your child feel in control of his or her allergies and also prepared for what to do in case of an attack. The best way to do this is to make it a commonly discussed topic, with conversations that range from educational to troubleshooting to reassurance.

Food-allergic children have to carry much of their own burdens, and it can be difficult for us as parents to watch them take on such an enormous responsibility at a young age. They are worried they might not survive and quickly become their own best advocates. Ours are the little ones who forgo nibbles, desserts, and snacks casually laid out at gatherings. Our kids are the ones too careful to relax all the way at a restaurant. These children see food differently than the cheery, unconcerned others who pop this or that hors d'oeuvre at an event without thinking twice. They are typically at the ready to avoid whatever food necessary from a fairly young age. There is a natural and healthy mourning process they go through as they begin to mature and come to realize the scope of the limitations necessary to successfully live with this medical condition.

After the initial tears have dried, the troops leap into action, often arms linked with their protective nonallergic siblings or best friends, to keep themselves safe from allergic reactions. It's touching to witness peers jump in. I remember just about every single one of my daughter's friends declaring loudly and proudly that they "don't even EAT nuts!" Yep, suddenly in solidarity with their soul sister, they actually "hate nuts!" emphatically. One slightly bewildered parent returned from a family vacation in Disneyland back to school and informed me that her son Miles was so concerned about his friend—my daughter—that he inquired before eating a nutty snack at the theme park, a plane ride away, whether it was safe and made sure to brush his teeth "extra good" that night. This was so that when he came home—several days later—he would not place his dear friend at risk. The empathy and simpatico from within the children's peer groups is lionhearted and strong and helps reinforce within our allergic children that as long as they are mindful, they can survive this.

Resources for Young Children

One of the great developments that has occurred as food allergies have burst into mainstream consciousness is the amount of tremendously vital resources available for elementary-school-age

children. With them at hand, it is easy to educate and encourage
your child. Here are some of my favorites.

Cloudy With a Chance of Meatballs (Movie)

My daughter and I were immersed in this fun and quirky comedic
children's movie at our local movie theater when out of the blue
one of the main characters had a peanut allergy and suffered an
allergic reaction as a notable plot point. This was the first time I'd
ever seen a scene in a children's movie with a food-allergic main
character. There are many cartoony elements in the scene that
make it unrealistic—it is an animated film about giant food, after
all—but suspending disbelief is one of the joys of moviegoing.
Our family thought it was a teachable moment for food allergies,
and we saw it twice.

Allie the Allergic Elephant by Nicole Smith (Picture Book)

This book is about an elephant who must avoid peanuts. Allie
must wear a special bracelet and keep a keen eye out for hidden
ingredients.

No Biggie Bunch by Heather Mehra and Kerry McManama (Picture Book Series)

The best part about these books is that they're written by parents
like us, for parents like us. They aren't written by the medical
community with the intention of helping patients; rather, this is
our own community's work supporting each other and speaking
a language we automatically understand. It's our own code, from

within our own tribe. This series is designed to help kids find ways to creatively cope with their food allergies.

Smart kids with various food allergies, Paige, Eliot, Scotty, Davis, and Greta, are best friends with Natalie, who has no food allergies. As a group, they're prepared with safe snacks and a ready response, and to them the social challenges of food allergies are "no biggie!" The books are plentiful and easy to find online and in bookstores. They explain the medical condition in a way that parents, teachers, and children can use to talk about allergies and help us all understand them better.

To Be a Nut or Not and *My Immune System Needs Glasses* by Michelle Nel Chow (Picture Books)

I find this author's description of her intention behind writing her books to be particularly inspiring:

> I began writing in hopes of providing a fun yet informative manner in which to share allergy information. My aspiration: to create books which would not only engage children with allergies but that might also be used as resources to aid in allergy education. For as challenging as it is navigating the world with anaphylactic allergies this journey has also has given our family, especially myself many gifts. We have our shifted focus from eating to doing. We are more aware of what equally is in our food as what is not. We have chosen to be more thankful for what life has given and not what we might do without. From unexpected friendships to becoming more empathetic people, Nolan's allergies have in fact given us many gifts.

Food Allergies Rock! by Kyle Dine
(Children's Music)

For your little music lovers and for parents alike, there's food allergy rock star Kyle Dine. Severely allergic and at risk for anaphylaxis himself with food allergies to peanut, tree nut, egg, seafood, and mustard, he rocks and rolls with a guitar that's lovingly named Ol' Betty. Kyle has made food allergies super cool for the younger set, with their own rock star who can relate completely to their experience by spreading his style of unique food allergy awareness and education through music. Kyle Dine invented the unique genre of "allergy musician" singlehandedly with a keen understanding that education is key. His main hit is called "Food Allergies Rock!" Kyle performs live in concerts all over the world and also at school assemblies. His show even includes the hilarious puppets EpiMan and EpiMan Jr. As he strums, he covers a range of helpful information about the most common food allergens, symptoms of a reaction, what an EpiPen is, and what to do in an emergency. Kyle Dine makes food allergies truly cool for our children. Here is his signature song.

"FOOD ALLERGIES ROCK!"

Written by Kyle Dine
Reprinted with Permission

(chorus)
Food Allergies Rock
Food Allergies Rock
To tell you the truth I would rather have them than not
Food Allergies Rock
Food Allergies Rock
I wouldn't trade them, I'm happy with what I got

Just a few things that I can't eat

But none of it is in my favorite treat

I can stay safe and I can stay well

Cuz I stay alert after the dinner bell

I could be a doctor or an astronaut

Whatever I choose I can reach the top

So I have food allergies

But I don't let them define me

Not to say that it's not tough

But I've had 'em so long I know enough

They make me special and that's why

I can walk around with my head held high

(chorus)

Preteens and Teenagers Need Your Help Staying Diligent

When your food-allergic children are itty-bitty, as difficult of an adjustment as it can be, they are largely with you, by your side, in your allergy-safe home or out with you or a trusted caregiver—usually with a support team of family surrounding them. Flash forward to a young, dating teen. Your support is every bit as needed, just in different ways.

Hardwired Changes

Teenagers can do some pretty outlandish things in our experienced, adult eyes, and while you might at first think this is because of peer pressure or willfulness, in fact it's primarily due to biology. Research shows that while their emotions have already matured, the rest hasn't fully matured yet—which is why teens don't have self-control and restraint. A lot of their basic teenage cognitive abilities, such as advanced reasoning, abstract thinking, and self-consciousness, rapidly expand during this time period. When adolescents are in the presence of peers, the reward circuitry in their brains is more activated compared with adults who are with their peers. These electrical signals impel us to seek pleasurable things, and it's only natural that such feelings are more intense in teens, susceptible as they are to social feedback, praise, and rejection—more so than adults. So teens often do what peers want them to do, or what they think peers want them to do, rather than what we might say is rational, and it's all in how they are hardwired.

Brain-mapping technologies show that the average teenager's brain looks slightly different from an adult's. The biggest differences are in the prefrontal cortex—a part of the brain associated with reasoning—and in the networks of brain cells that link the cortex to regions of the brain that are less about reasoning and thinking and more about emotion. So when teens turn about fifteen or sixteen years old, many of their brain cells in the cortex decrease—a process called "synaptic pruning," explains noted Yale psychiatrist Dr. Michel Jean-Baptiste. While other cells are created, new connections form among them, so teenagers— eventually, as they mature—are left with just the right number and balance of synaptic connections later in life. Dr. Jean-Baptiste further explains about the lack of maturation in the fiber tracts, which are connected but lag behind just the frontal and prefrontal cortex and comprises the emotional part of the brain. Those pathways continue to mature throughout our lives, but it's new development that places our teenagers in a very precarious situation: The emotions have already matured but the rest hasn't fully matured, which is why teens don't have self-control and restraint yet.

Risky Behavior

Unfortunately, this risk-taking behavior means teens are at the highest risk for food-induced anaphylactic reactions. Some teens engage in risky behaviors like not reading labels, knowingly—horrifyingly—eating foods that could contain their allergen, or not carrying emergency medicine when they are out with friends. The level of risk they take depends on their social circumstances and how they perceive dangers. Some teens don't want to be different and carry their auto-injectors, and some fail to take their potentially lifesaving medication along when engaging in certain activities or if they are wearing tight clothing. Some teens don't tell their friends about their food allergies and would prefer for the school to do it. Understandably, they want their friends to know that they have a food allergy and about food allergies in general, but they want someone else to educate them. Other teens have an easier time managing their food allergies and something that is akin to body integrity.

Ways You Can Support Teenagers

Even though they are gaining independence, teenagers need extra help staying diligent. Effects of allergies can range from annoying to debilitating to life-threatening. Your teen knows it's not just annoying itchy eyes and hives—allergies can be life-threatening. They just need as many practical tools for navigating this fact as the two of you can brainstorm. Here are some suggestions.

Conversation

Encourage open communication and be sure to let your teen know that you are open to all of his or her questions and want to know how he or she is feeling. Provide teens a period of amnesty in your conversations, and allow them to share with you about "rule breaking" without any risk of punishment. If you're careful but calm, your teen will have the added advantage of a good role model and can approach his or her allergies with wisdom instead of worry.

Carrying Medication Is Nonnegotiable, So Make It Fun

Teens have to be taught to be consistent in carrying their medication: Make this a nonnegotiable family rule. Teens that appear reluctant may feel better if they get a carrying case that appeals to their personal style; different auto-injector carriers may help teens feel more relaxed because they allow them to keep epinephrine with them in a less-conspicuous way. They need a reasonable method to motivate them to keep the pens on their person; this can be a woman's purse or carryall purse. Older boys, outside of school backpacks, like to put everything in their pockets, so it must fit comfortably. Realistically, teens don't want to stand out for any reason, and they certainly don't want to have something that looks like an "old lady" fanny pack strapped around their waists.

Planning for Outings with Friends

Empower your teen to take an active role in managing his or her food allergy by helping your teen to plan, behind the scenes, for social situations. For example, gather menus from popular restaurants. Encourage your teen to practice making good choices and informing restaurant staff about food allergies. Then call ahead to find out about safe options in advance. You could also brainstorm together about how to handle tricky situations, like creating "chef cards" to hand to a waiter that explains the allergy fully. Try to be as concrete and literal as you are able: Problem solve or role play with your teenagers about exactly how, and precisely where, they will carry their emergency medication.

Instilling Confidence

Make sure your teen feels comfortable suggesting restaurants that are good choices for him or her and is willing to speak up if a restaurant is a risky choice. Go out with your teens and encourage them to practice talking about their food allergies with waiters, chefs, and restaurant managers so that when they inevitably go out to eat with friends, they can stay safe.

Encourage Teens to Have Their Own Open Conversations

Ideally, your teen would talk to everyone he or she knows about his or her food allergies. Making food allergies a common talking point in everyday relationships among teens means everyone knows what the allergy is, how to respond if a reaction happens, and what foods friends need to avoid if they want to spend time with you. Teaching friends about epinephrine auto-injectors and showing them how to properly inject epinephrine if there is an allergic reaction is commonplace now. Instill in them the necessity to teach their friends—especially chocolate-bearing suitors— to read all labels before buying your teens any tasty treats. Special holiday or bite-size candies can have different ingredients than their traditional versions, so teens have to be helped and taught to keep their eyes wide open when purchasing gifts.

Making Use of Smartphones

Initially, and understandably, food-allergic teenagers might be nervous about dining out without their parents and may forget what to ask or what to order. Having a smartphone, tablet, or other mobile device in hand, with valuable information about specific venues, possible food choices, and online menus at their fingertips, is useful and makes dining out easier for social, busy teenagers.

During dining experiences on her own with friends or on a date, my own teenager, Charlotte, occasionally finds it helpful and reassuring to snap pictures of food labels and text them to me from her iPhone for a speedy yet discreet second opinion. You can compile lists about their allergies right on their phones in a "Notes" section so they can refer back to this information as needed, since it's readily available and at their fingertips. These lists can include questions to ask at restaurants, information to share about peanut and tree nut aliases, hidden sources, and other key materials.

Train Closest Friends and Dating Interests for Emergencies

EpiPens come with handy training devices that mimic the real deal. The EpiPen training device is easily distinguishable from the real auto-injector, as the label clearly states "Training Device" and is pale blue. It functions in the same way as the real EpiPen but does not contain a needle or epinephrine. Encourage your teen to ask those closest to him or her to practice, practice,

practice. Then, if an emergency arises, they will know what to do in the seconds that can make all the difference.

Apps for Preteens and Teens

A great app can help make life with allergies a bit easier. We live in an "appy world," with several mobile applications available to manage our day-to-day activities. With rapidly evolving technology, managing food allergies has become easier, and plenty of these apps are cool enough to motivate your teen. There are apps that can scan product bar codes, link to emergency services, display ingredients and what is in your food, show you how to administer epinephrine, and identify safe food options when you're traveling or away from home.

Depending on your preference and what type of smartphone your teenager has, options abound for food allergy apps. Plenty of them are completely free of charge and can easily be downloaded. Here are some good ones to check out.

Fooducate

This app was created by dietitians and concerned parents. It has an ever-growing database of over 200,000 unique products in the United States that informs your teen about Big 8 allergens in foods. It also provides gluten information. Plus, it offers suggestions for safe alternatives. Here's how it works: Your savvy preteen or teen can scan a product UPC bar code, search for products, or browse by categories and get a complete nutritional analysis.

The First Aid App by American Red Cross

This is available for download at no cost and offers step-by-step, easy-to-understand information about what to do when you are having an allergic reaction. It can connect your teen immediately with 911, so first aid is available anytime, anywhere.

WhyRiskIt?

This food allergy education app was in fact created by a teenager. Nineteen-year-old Nick Pothier designed the app with the hope that it would provide easy-to-access information for teens with allergies so that they can be safer and take significantly fewer risks. It features lifesaving information that should be on the fingertips of every allergic teen, such as signs and symptoms of anaphylaxis and treatment and emergency procedures.

AllergyEats

This app helps identify restaurants where the local food allergy community in an area has had positive and safe experiences.

Unique Challenges in Dating

When I was a teenager (to quote my daughter's mathematics instructor, "back when the Earth was still coalescing"), there were no food-labeling laws in place. So, when I was out and about, I was right on the numbers, and a quarter of the time I was eating, I succumbed to severe allergic reactions—sometimes multiple times during the course of a week. The pitfalls of dating and dining out lurked everywhere; most attempts at going on a date at a restaurant ended with a trip to the emergency room due to cross-contamination.

Encourage Them to Apply Their Knowledge

Nowadays, awareness and advocacy are at an all-time high. What seemed impossible when I was a teen is now the standard. From fast-food joints to college cafeterias and everywhere in between, our teens have the benefit of guidelines in place to ensure that they can know, down to the last drop, what's in their food. If your teenager can keep his or her mind together, even when spun a bit by romance, there are more options available.

Make Disclosure a Prerequisite

Teens are socially tight-knit and are more likely to date someone in their close circle of friends, so if everyone knows, then there are no surprises when friendships blossom into relationships. If your teen has prepared his or her friends, then perhaps someone he or she chooses to date is already informed. If not, encourage your teen to talk to the person about allergies as soon as possible. As difficult or embarrassing as this may seem to teens, they are forced to have an open and honest conversation with their boyfriends or girlfriends about their food allergies. Help them feel comfortable sharing their concerns, depending on the severity of their allergy, as this will no doubt aid them in making their new beaus more comfortable as well. It's important for them to honestly note warning signs that their interest isn't up for the challenge. If a suitor can't forgo the Reese's Peanut Butter Cups at the movies with a peanut-allergic beloved, he or she is not ready to be in a relationship with your teen.

Hand-holding, Hugging, and Kissing

Dating is a rite of passage in middle school and high school and a means of growth and coming of age, but it can also be a dizzying game of Russian roulette if food-allergic teens aren't prepared for intimate touch. Hand-holding, hugging, and kissing can pass food allergens from one person to another, increasing the risk of reaction.

Teens fall in love, and everything they've learned about food allergies can suddenly disappear from their mind when their date leans forward for that kiss. But when they have food allergies, the harsh reality is that even the smallest amount of residue can lead to anaphylaxis and death. One researcher has suggested that patients with peanut allergy benefit from counseling regarding the risks of kissing or sharing utensils—even if a partner has brushed his or her teeth or chewed gum. Advice to reduce risks, although not as ideal as total avoidance, includes waiting a few hours and eating a subsequent peanut-free meal. Teens who don't want to talk to their parents about this can instead talk to their doctor about what makes the most sense for their particular allergic situation.

Many teens and young adults tell us that their significant others avoid the allergy-causing food on days when they will be hanging out together. Mercifully, others say their boyfriends or girlfriends have cut the allergen out of their diets entirely.

Teach your teen to plan ahead if he or she, ahem, plans on action! As tricky and uncomfortable as this part of the conversation might be for us parents, make sure you've taught your teens to be open with their boyfriends and girlfriends before going in for the kiss. Their dates need to have been vigilant and conscious of their food choices that day, have washed their hands and face, have thoroughly brushed their teeth and flossed. It's better safe than sorry with teens (with, let's face it, other overwhelming concerns to their health and well-being), and if they can be co-erced into getting in the habit of a squeaky-clean, allergy-safe mouth, it's one less concern for your teen. One teen tip: Keep a special, travel-size "safe" toothbrush in your medical bag that a date can use. This would have been my number one top tip back when I was dating, if someone had shared it with me.

Activities

If a romantic interest wants to prepare a romantic dinner for your teen or is making reservations at your local bistro, he or she must be taught how to take extra precautions to ask for help at the grocery store or how to have a conversation with the chef or waiter to ensure that anything being prepared does not contain the al-lergen. This includes cross-contamination. Taking these pre-date steps not only shows how to care for each other but also sets them up for an evening uninterrupted by an allergic attack.

Teens can also try to move the focus of their dates away from food. There are movies, plays, concerts, hikes up mountains, or fun group trips to bowling alleys. Activities abound where your teen will be safe.

The More Everyone Knows the Drill, the More Fun Can Be Had

Managing friendships, romance, and food allergies is only an ob-stacle if you make it into one. If your teen brings his or her med-icine and is prepared and everyone is aware, then the focus can be primarily on the joys of being young, hanging out, and dating. Perhaps the most important thing teens can hear is your assur-ance that they can relax, enjoy, and have fun!

6

Help
from the
Whole Family

DESPITE THE DIFFICULTY of managing food allergies, our indomitable human spirit shines through, and with ingenuity and mutual respect, we parents are doing our best to help our families, ourselves, and each other. Food allergy dad and Food Allergy Alliance of the Mid-South support group founder Billy Barnett shares,

> I had very little knowledge of food allergies. I thought a food allergy resulted in an upset stomach or skin rash if someone ate the wrong food. I had never heard of anaphylaxis or that someone could die from an allergic reaction. It was a strange feeling. We mostly felt shocked, but also experienced a lot of confusion. How can food that is supposed to nourish our bodies, that people eat every day, be almost like poison to our son's body? My biggest dream is that someday my son will grow out of his allergies or scientists find a cure in his lifetime. Regardless, my hope is that he lives as normal a life as any other child. And in that normal life we can keep him safe and that he never feels singled out

in a negative way, bullied or a burden to anyone. I hope we can teach him confidence in managing his allergies safely and teach him to assert himself as needed. Learning and navigating our food allergy journey has taught our family compassion, perseverance and patience. I hope my sons use those characteristics to bless others in their lives.

Gather Everyone's Support During the Challenging Transition Days

No doubt, everyone was used to the household being one way. And now so much will be different. One of the best ways to successfully navigate the early days of transitioning into the new lifestyle of strict avoidance is to get everybody on board. From grandparents to cousins to siblings, the whole family can come together because if they understand why such changes are necessary, making them happen will come that much more easily. Here are some things everyone needs to understand during the inevitable period of adjustment as everyone gets used to a new way of life. Explain to the whole family that, for the time being, you all might need to take extra cautious steps to keep a food-allergic child safe while parents and caregivers work hard to establish some safe, allergenic perimeters. This can mean any of the following:

- Going out to eat at restaurants may be postponed for a while.
- An upcoming vacation may have to be delayed.
- Parties, play dates, and sporting events might be put on the back burner right now.
- Food and menu changes around the house will be essential.
- Favorite foods and snacks may not be served for a while, or at all.

- Even favorite lotions, soaps, and shampoos might have
  to change.

Look for the Joys Along the Way

In the introduction, I described the story of my own daughter at
her very distant, safe school when she was younger and the long
journey I took each day. I slowly adjusted to my daily commute
across the Golden Gate Bridge to find the balance I needed to
survive. Human connection helps so much, and so does finding
nourishing ways to uplift the journey. One time on my commute,
a fancy cruise ship straight out of *The Love Boat* eased up and
underneath the bridge, and about 400 people below, all on the
deck of the boat, called up to me, waving. I braked, stopped
suddenly in the middle of the bridge, and saluted the sea-bound
with their vastly different vantage point. We all did, we-the-mad-
commuters. Just this once, all the frantic whizzing, commuting,
driving ceased. Frozen in a moment, we ground to a halt. It was
a still moment. No one honked. We could clearly see each other's
faces, who was wearing glasses, who had grown a goatee, who
wore braces. That close. Some people on the boat were laughing,
others got teary—it was surprisingly intimate to see each other
in this way, each of us on our own travel, going somewhere and
elsewhere. Some ocean people flashed peace signs, grinning from
ear to ear, some whistled and catcalled up the bridge, some
placed hands over their hearts and sang out to us, but everyone
acknowledged each other, each of us.

I waved happily back out the window until my elbow hurt, and
my cheeks were sore from grinning so hard without even realiz-
ing. I waved until they cruised all the way underneath and began
to disappear away from us, off to some luxurious other location.

Then we all just started up our cars again, driving onward to wherever we were headed—me to my nut-allergic daughter. Moments like this, which I would not otherwise experience, have enriched my journey so that I can enjoy each step and every moment for what it is.

Mothers Unite

A large group of stay-at-home moms have already swiftly taken to blogging and the Internet and have formed an impromptu food allergy community based on organically homegrown grassroots "support groups," sometimes right from our kitchen tables. Empowered with the engagement and support of our community at large, busy on chat boards advocating for increased knowledge and awareness of food allergies nationally and at the community level, food allergy mothers have been dubbed and anointed "Mama Bears" by online media worldwide. There's "Allergy Schmallergy," a cheery website with insights and even cooking tips; humor often plays a role in coping with food allergies. Having carried our children in our own wombs for such a long duration, we already have an innate sense of our babies and particularly the nonverbal cues that we share back and forth. As moms, we tend to never underestimate the power of our intuition for our little creatures, we can often sense danger, and we can tell with a quick look if something isn't quite right with our children. This is a useful skill when navigating the road of life with food allergies.

Fathers Mobilize

There are countless food allergy fathers like Billy Barnett, all of whom care deeply about their kids, and there are many ways to express love and caring that don't fit into a conventional box deemed this way or that way by society at large. Most dads say they knew in an instant that their lives would never be the same when they learned that their child had been diagnosed with food allergies. More than one dad has described the diagnosis as something that made them feel powerless, and others admitted they were angry. Quite a combination! It explains, perhaps, why food allergy dads are particularly helpful in advocating for their young ones: They seem particularly adept at converting that initial powerlessness and anger into an indomitable driving force.

Sometimes poor communication with moms, or even their own childhood experiences, can prevent dads from connecting as deeply with their children. Child development is part of a complex social system that varies widely from family to family, and there is no single right way for fathers to be involved. Research has found that the value of father involvement is determined by the quality of the interaction between fathers and their children—for example, a father's responsiveness to the needs of his child—rather than the amount of time fathers spend with their children. All dads at all income levels and in all sorts of families—for example, food-allergic homes with two dads—may at times feel isolated, vulnerable, and painfully left out of the social fray that mothers can easily engulf themselves in. Dads and father figures offer our families extra strength, a strong shoulder to cry on, an arm on a shoulder at the ball game. I learned so much from my own father as a food-allergic person, and I am still learning from him daily. Fathers' presence and involvement is as crucial to children's healthy development as mothers'. Experiencing validation of their importance in the general parenting literature has made fathers much more conscious of their value and, in turn, led to their greater desire to be involved. So, rather than deferring to moms to be in charge of the family food allergies, it's great for dads to participate on every level and get involved in advocacy.

Taking Care of Ourselves
to Take Care of Our Allergic One

Not surprisingly, we experience significant anxiety about keeping our children safe from allergenic foods and yet are equally concerned about the possible negative repercussions of parental hypervigilance or helicoptering around our young kids in our best effort to keep them safe from their food allergies and the dire consequences that can befall our families. The best way to strike the right balance is to be sure to acknowledge our own feelings and to take care of ourselves.

As parents, we can sometimes experience strong emotions when our children have a chronic medical condition. Intellectually we know it isn't rational, but we can be plagued with the feelings as we see our children struggle for normalcy. These emotions are complicated and conflicting and can cause difficulties between friends, relatives, and even spouses. Here are some of the main feelings that can accompany having a child with a chronic food allergy.

Denial: This is an important coping mechanism when reality is too frightening, overwhelming, or perceived as too much of a threat to our sense of control. It can be a form of natural protection, but over time it should be alleviated to allow us to discuss our fears and develop a strong food allergy action plan. This can be effectively handled by a professional who has expertise in the stress of surviving and thriving with a family member's medical condition.

Anger: We can become overcome by anger in a matter of seconds when we enviously see another family with their children and how easy it all looks for them, or we might resent the food allergy diagnosis and all the limitations it suddenly places on the family as a whole. When we see a news story about someone who has succumbed to his or her food allergy due to incompetence or an accident, how can we not feel the rush of fury? Rather than trying to avoid the anger—because outwardly some people show anger more than others, but almost no one is never angry—learn instead to express it in healthy ways. There are better biological releases than just snapping, and you can feel this complicated emotion and still be an amazing parent.

Guilt: You may feel guilty that you hadn't noticed symptoms sooner or the nagging feeling that you yourself are healthy while your child is so restricted by his or her diet. The dictionary defines guilt as the feeling of responsibility that follows an offense. However, with food allergies, remind yourself that no offense has been committed, no one is responsible for the food allergy. Since you have done nothing wrong, it will greatly affect your quality of life to punish yourself. Reminding yourself and your family members that you are not guilty, and repeating it to each other often, can help to dispel and calm these feelings, and if that fails, you can seek professional help to adjust to this aspect of food allergy life.

Anxiety: Caregiving takes a considerable emotional toll because you need to gather up your own strength and try to do so with a smile. It's tough to watch anyone go through an illness, but the emotional toll of this chronic condition with unpredictable allergic reactions is extremely difficult, and these reactions create a sense of urgency, chaos, and confusion for us. It suddenly feels like nothing is in our control anymore as we waver from hoping for the best to fearing the worst. Get centered, get answers, and get support so you don't feel isolated with these natural feelings, because you can't drive a car on an empty gas tank. We need to make sure there is an element of self-care firmly in place to reduce anxiety.

Exhaustion: Extreme tiredness makes even routine tasks difficult, but when you add in the needed vigilance to read every food label every time and to diligently carry epinephrine all the time, it's easy to feel tired and run down. The demands of caring for a sick child can be downright overwhelming. Caring for yourself and resting from time to time is just as important as your child's food allergy because when you reach that point of fatigue, both you and your child are impacted. You can start to catch every cold and flu that's going around, or you may wake after a night of sleep still feeling very tired. Remember, you can't always carve out the extra time for sleep, but you can always, always get more happiness and hope for yourself! Make yourself laugh, find mini ways to pamper yourself, prioritize activities that bring enjoyment, and most of all take a break to maintain personal relationships. And when someone offers to help so you can take a short break—let them.

Protecting Your Marriage

Marital tensions and conflict can arise due to differences in parenting philosophy and practice. Mothers and fathers sometimes have differing opinions regarding the measures needed to protect the child, even a perfectly healthy offspring, but now add allergic reactions and it's easy to see where differing opinions and various issues arise. There are no absolutes, but some moms might tend to shelter children from the smallest possibility of risk whereas some dads desire to expand their child's life experiences as much as possible. Or perhaps it's the other way around: a careful and cautious father and a mother who wants to celebrate each moment with junior *con gusto*. However, either scenario has the same end result: Food allergies have an effect on quality of spouse life. Here our food allergy dad Billy Barnett offers a message about marriage:

> Most people that I talk to have never heard about food allergies or what can happen during a reaction. I think it is natural for Moms to take on the lead role of protecting her child when diagnosed, but Dads have that same responsibility. We need to know how to read labels; we need to be able to clearly communicate their emergency care plan to schools and babysitters; we need to be just as involved in their care. Parenting takes a team, especially when your children have special needs.

It Feels Good to Change the World

When we are working to change the world, we don't feel nearly as helpless. Our sense of mission and devotion to our children can drive us to work to make the world a safer place for them. It also helps us to stay motivated, be inexhaustible, and feel powerful.

Fund-raising

FARE, the world's largest nonprofit organization dedicated to food allergy awareness, education, research, and advocacy, mobilizes families from state to state and even city to city for annual walkathons, complete with prizes and festivities surrounding the events, which take place in communities nationwide. The fund-raising efforts make a huge difference in our lives, helping reach the next step to find the cure and make the world a safer place for us. There are live music and vendors galore (all allergy-friendly and safe), and teams strive to acknowledge and support food-allergic family and friends. These events unite thousands and thousands of people, with the shared goal of ensuring a safer world for all of us who live with food allergies and are searching for a cure.

Changing Laws

Some parents lobby for auto-injectors in schools, for example, by heading all the way to Congress; others fight for increased safety measures to help not only their children but all children with food allergies.

Awareness Events

After tragically losing his teen son to a peanut allergy on a family vacation to celebrate graduation, one incredible Bay Area dad organized his own full-scale, annual Food Allergy Walk-A-Thon. He even solicited corporate sponsorships and local sports heroes to honor his basketball-loving son.

Making Activity Environments Safe

I recently received a correspondence from a food allergy dad who had contacted the local sports arena and arranged for a peanut-free zone so families could come out together and cheer on our Golden State Warriors despite peanut allergies. Fortunately, this has turned into an annual event, with several clusters of dates so many can enjoy the experience, and the concept of safe, designated areas for live sports viewing has begun to spread from state to state.

Blogging

Parents are devoted to their children, and many have found their own voices and their own heartfelt, rich stories to share. Blogging is one way parents can spread the word and also take action. Smart food allergy management strategies and connecting with others who are managing food allergies every day can help us all feel more in control and alleviate some of the stress. Parents bring many unique ideas and a fresh perspective to food allergy awareness and advocacy.

One blogger, known simply by his avatar Food Allergy Dad, has made it his personal mission since 2012 to inspire positive attitudes to food and life in everyone affected by food allergies. His blog profile provides a warm introduction of "a man who, after a life-changing couple of years, decided to dedicate himself to bringing more positivity into the lives of people affected by severe food allergies."

Another amazing blogger, Mocha Dad, discusses on his website how his initial confusion turned to action. He writes with honesty about his own experience and dedicates his writings with a mission: "One Father's Quest to Be a Better Dad." A dinner trip to the Olive Garden with his family and young daughter was the beginning of his food allergy journey. He urges parents to always carry an EpiPen, yet encourages families to still try dining out and to try new things with vigilance.

The Perils and Wonders of Household Pets

Parents of kids with food allergies have the challenge of teaching our children—often from a very young age—to manage a chronic health condition while maintaining a positive attitude and a sense of normalcy. A family pet is a welcome addition to a household and helps to teach children responsibility (albeit with additional work for Mom and Dad—typically after much bargaining and negotiating promises to the contrary!).

Beware of Allergy to the Pet

According to the Asthma and Allergy Foundation of America (AAFA), at least 15 percent of Americans who have allergies are allergic to pets, and adults who fall into this group are also more likely to have children with similar conditions. AAFA figures show that as many as seven out of ten children will develop pet allergies if both parents are affected. However, it's also entirely possible for children to develop allergies when both parents are allergy-free.

Sometimes it's easy to pinpoint the root cause of your child's allergic reactions, and sometimes it's not. Signs of a potential pet allergy in children can include runny nose; sneezing; red or watery eyes; itching; and in more severe cases, rashes, hives, and even the development of full-blown asthma. There are, however, other allergens, such as mold, that can create almost identical symptoms. So how can you tell if pets are the cause? First consider whether your children have ever been exposed to animals, and if so, whether they have exhibited any subsequent reactions. Symptoms of a pet allergy usually show up within thirty minutes or so after contact but sometimes can take as long as eight to twelve hours to surface.

Even if there's no pet in the family home, pet allergies can cause lots of problems for children who will be around animals when they're out and about or visiting the homes of relatives and friends. The truth is, pesky allergens from warm-blooded animals can cause problems for kids and parents alike. When your household pet licks itself, the saliva gets on its fur or feathers. As the saliva dries, protein particles become airborne and work their way into fabrics in the home.

Cats are the worst offenders because the protein from their saliva is extremely tiny and they tend to lick themselves more than other animals as part of grooming. Of course, not all animals will trigger an allergic reaction. While some kids are more allergic to cats or dogs, the allergy can range to hamsters, guinea pigs, birds, and on and on. Fur and feathers can create allergic symptoms or asthmatic episodes in our children with allergies. The fact is, all breeds have the potential to cause an allergic reaction in your child—even fancy hybrids; there's really no truly allergy-free type of cat, dog, or bird.

When my daughter was little and seemingly allergic to everything on the planet, we asked her pediatrician exasperatedly, what kind of pet could she have? Even borrowing the bunny mascot from her pre-school for scheduled, calendared, forty-eight-hour weekend visits caused nosebleeds. What was our beloved pediatrician's flat, well-meaning—albeit unimaginative—response? "Try a turtle." (Fine. We did.)

If your newly found food allergy intuition gives you a hunch that a new family addition is suddenly causing allergic reactions, your best option is to confirm the diagnosis immediately to be certain and to rule out that it's not something else newly introduced into your home environment. If a doctor determines that your son or daughter definitely has severe pet allergies, the easiest course of action is to prevent contact with the animal, which could mean finding a great new home for your pet. Your family's and of course your child's attachment to a beloved, dear sweet pet makes this an understandably heartbreaking decision. Nonetheless, it's probably the best thing to do for your child's health. When explaining the circumstances, you can try to remind your child of how important it is to remain healthy. It also may be useful to ask your pediatrician or allergist for advice on how to best approach the discussion. In the interim, while you search for a new home for your pet, it's ideal to not allow the animal into or near the allergic child's bedroom. However, absolutely, you can lovingly visit often, replenish water and food supplies, and generally check in. If feasible, it could be best to keep the pet out of the house entirely if an enclosed and safe backyard area is available and the weather permits. Either way, since dander gets tracked into the house on the soles of shoes and even on clothes and hands, it's a good idea to wash and clean frequently to get rid of all allergenic particles and eliminate hair and dust. Bathe your pet frequently, the more often the better—the Humane Society's official recommendation is weekly washing of a pet to reduce allergic reactions by 84 percent. Although a last resort, it is conceivable that children could be given allergy treatments, from allergy shots and nose sprays to antihistamine pills, but pragmatically and realistically, it's significantly easier to find a welcome new nonallergic spot for Fido.

Time also plays a factor, as children might outgrow pet allergies (my allergic daughter did!). Meanwhile, watch out for allergic reactions in your home and when visiting the homes of your friends and families with pets. Your kids will also come in contact with animals around your neighborhood and in petting zoos. Although risk of allergen exposure might be low outside of your home, considering these contacts and ways to minimize risk of allergen exposure is helpful. For example, be certain that your child's hands are cleaned after contact with animal saliva if he or she visits a petting zoo before hands go in the mouth, eyes, or nose.

Watch Out for Pet Food

This is only one half of the equation: while a nuisance and uncomfortable, pet dander allergies aren't the only consideration in an allergic household. Even if your allergic or anaphylactic child can handle the doggiest dog dander all over your house, it's essential to stay vigilant and mindful of hidden allergens contained in your pet's food because plenty contain Big 8 allergens and ingredients. Common ingredients in pet meals and treats are dairy, wheat, and soy. Also look for peanuts, fish, shellfish, egg, and all potential allergens. The ingredients used will vary depending on the animal being fed (dogs, cats, rodents, birds, fish, reptiles, etc.).

Also, keep in mind that labeling can be a bit tricky, as the law governing it does not apply to pet food. If you are looking for specific food allergens and have any questions after reading the label, call the manufacturer to ask. For toddlers and little ones who are still putting objects in their mouths and possibly eating things that they find on the floor, direct ingestion of the pet food will need to be prevented.

When thinking about allergens in pet food, consider ways that your child could come in contact with the pet food. Food allergens can be transferred via saliva. There are peanuts and whey, a milk derivative, found in birdseed; egg is present in most puppy foods and kitten kibbles; and peanut butter or salmon often lurk inside store-bought dog bones and even latex chewy toys. It's only natural that your child will come into frequent contact with the pet's food from just basic general contact with your furry family member, from being licked and nuzzled by your pet or from handling and serving up the food itself.

What you'll need to stay on track with your allergy food sleuthing is a food allergy pet strategy. First, familiarize yourself with the complete listing of derivative names for each and every allergen you must avoid in the various kibbles and chows. Even without the FALCPA labeling on pet food labels, however, you can check for voluntary warnings on domestic animal food packaging because some products will thoughtfully contain advisory statements indicating that the product is made on equipment or in facilities that produce other products containing peanuts or tree nuts, wheat, and some other allergens.

Common Allergens in Pet Foods and Their Derivative Names

You will need to keep an eye out for hidden allergens in your pet's food. Here are other, less common, names of Big 8 allergens:

- **Milk:** butter esters, casein, caseinates, casein hydrolysate, diacetyl, ghee, lactalbumin, lactalbumin phosphate, lactoferrin lactose, lactulose, rennet casein, tagatose, whey, whey protein hydrolysate
- **Egg:** albumin, globulin, lecithin, lysozyme, meringue, ovalbumin, vitellin
- **Wheat:** durum, farina, seitan, semolina, spelt, triticale, wheatgrass
- **Soy:** hydrolyzed protein, isolate, kinnoko flour, miso, lecithin, natto, soya, tamari, tempeh, texturized vegetable protein (TVP), tofu, yuba
- **Fish:** caviar, kosher gelatin, marine gelatin, omega-3, Worcestershire sauce
- **Shellfish:** cockle, crawdad, krill, langoustine, limpet
- **Peanuts:** arachis, arachis hypogaea, arachnic oil, goober peas, hypogaeic acid, nut "meats"
- **Tree Nuts:** castanea, carya, fagus, ginkgo, juglans, lychee, pigñoli, pili, praline, shea

When in doubt, you should always place a phone call directly to the manufacturer or hit the Internet and thoroughly review the ingredient section of the website listed on the pet food product, if available, to confirm the source of all of the various vitamins and proteins. Interestingly, it should be noted that your pet, itself, can develop and suffer from food allergies. Dogs and cats can have signs and symptoms that sometimes look common or that might be attributed to something else. Pet itching and scratching are high on the list, with odor, ear infections, skin infections, and surface bumps, to name a few symptoms. You can talk to your veterinarian if your allergic home now has a seemingly allergic pet. Laboratory tests surprisingly similar to the ones used for us help make the diagnosis of allergies in your domestic animal.

The Benefits of Having a Pet

It's not by coincidence that it is very common for pet owners to describe their furry friend as a part of the family. Pets are reported to enhance the quality of family life in numerous ways, including minimizing tension between family members and helping them to develop increased compassion for living things.

If a clean bill of health has been established by your allergist for one and all in the household, the great news is that it's been well proven that pets can boost our spirits—research has repeatedly illustrated this over the years. Psychological studies have also demonstrated a direct and concrete link between pet ownership and improved self-esteem in children. Pets apparently help children develop empathy and improve their cognitive abilities. Furthermore, pets have enormous health benefits for people and have been shown to lower blood pressure, improve recovery from heart disease, and even reduce rates of asthma and allergy in children who grow up with them in the house. Domestic animals also serve as a great natural antidepressant—research has shown that petting them can increase the release of endorphins and other chemicals in the body that are linked with pleasure.

The relationship between food allergies and anxiety is complicated: allergies are an immunological health problem, and anxiety is a mental health issue, but the two seem to have a strong link, both directly and indirectly. There's the fear of having allergic reactions, and since allergies are caused by an inadequate immune system response, the additional stress on your immune system only makes it work less efficiently, resulting in more serious allergy symptoms than if you did not have stress. One of the reasons for the therapeutic effects of domestic animals is that they fulfill our basic human need for touch, and so the correlation between pets and happiness seems undeniable. Having the love and companionship of a loyal companion can make your son or daughter feel important and help him or her develop a positive self-image, and a pet can add unconditional love and deep joy to your family's life by increasing exercise and providing companionship, and even structure and routine, for an unpredictable food allergy lifestyle.

7

Ensuring
Sibling Support

WHEN A FAMILY has one child diagnosed with food allergies, the questions pour forth: Will my severely food-allergic child's brothers and sisters also have food allergies? Or with one severely allergic child, will my next baby be born with food allergies? Will a younger sibling who seems just fine now develop food allergies? We want to know what to anticipate, and it can feel as though there are more questions floating around than there are answers. First things first: You need to prepare your other children for a change in lifestyle.

Talking to the Siblings of a Food-Allergic Child

Gather all of your children together and first deliver the good news: While this is an undeniable blow, with a period of adjustment ahead, the future still looks bright for your family. Now, at last, there is an explanation and a diagnosis for their brother's or sister's rapid onset of illness and symptoms—which had been unpredictable until now. A scary trip to the emergency room may have preceded the allergist's findings, but today there is actual, definitive news about how to keep brother or sister safe. There will be a new normal, but finally there will be more balance and predictability—family life will become less panicked by a suddenly-ill and suffering young family member.

It will require lifestyle changes that might seem confusing at first but will begin to make more sense as you all steer together out of the constant danger zone. Honestly explain to all of the children together why it is necessary to develop and agree on these action plans:

- Emergency responses
- Safe foods at home and outside the home
- Establishing a safe family lifestyle that eliminates allergens

Do impress the fact that their sibling's allergic reactions have serious consequences, and while this may seem scary, the children can all work together to protect each other.

Turning Lifestyle Changes into Valuable Teachable Moments

Allergic families think a lot about food—logically and literally, we have to. One of the benefits of a food-allergic lifestyle is an awareness and interest in everything that goes into our mouths and a desire not to take chances with frivolous munching. Instead, we think about nourishment in a thoughtful and contemplative way, examining the whole food item and seeking to understand the genesis of everything we consume. Parents can take this food allergy crisis and turn it into opportunity: Here is a realistic life lesson for our children that can lead to robust health and wise, lifelong eating choices and habits, regardless of whether or not a child outgrows his or her food allergy.

Siblings need to be encouraged to partner together and provide additional support in the home, as this is a shared family experience. That means mealtimes become more than just times to eat. Instead, they evolve into meaningful times to help one another out and make each other feel comfortable.

Research Insights from Twins

Twins provide an insight into households with multiple allergies. Bay Area wife and mother Missy, now a grown woman with children of her own, was born an identical twin. Missy and her twin sister share a fingerprint so similar that the difference is unable to be discerned by the naked eye. They are both food allergic, yet each has vastly different food allergies! Missy is anaphylactically allergic to tree nuts, and her sister can tolerate tree nuts perfectly well but is severely allergic to avocados, which Missy can safely eat free of any symptoms. Twin studies at hospitals across the country are currently examining these food allergy findings in clinical trials in the hopes of uncovering answers to many food allergy riddles. It's fascinating to peek into the immunological differences between siblings so closely tied together.

Twin zygosity is the genetic relationship of twins. There are two types of twins: monozygotic twins, or identical twins—like Missy and her mirror-image twin sister—and dizygotic twins, also known as fraternal twins. Identical twins have exactly identical DNA strands; they are the same sex and have very similar physical traits. They come from one egg that is fertilized by one sperm. At some point in time after conception, the egg splits, resulting in two babies. Fraternal twins only have half-identical DNA; that is, only one strand of the double-stranded DNA is the same. They come from two individual eggs that are fertilized by two individual sperms. The Mt. Sinai School of Medicine has gone so far as to claim that genetics accounts for 81.6 percent of the risk of peanut allergy, but its studies haven't made a substantive claim about the other Big 8 yet. Overall, the results are not exact, but one thing that many twin studies have in common is that they have uncovered and agree that allergies among identical twins, who have identical DNA strands, are shared more often than allergies among fraternal twins, who have only one strand of DNA in common.

Could Another Sibling Develop an Allergy?

A common, natural question parents and siblings ask at this time is whether there is an increased risk of a sibling also developing a food allergy. Even with all of the data, there's nothing preventative to date that can be done in advance to prevent food allergies in siblings. Despite all of the current studies, there is no evidence, practical, scientific, or otherwise, that says this is possible.

There are plenty of households where our children have multiple allergies—to the Big 8 and beyond—among various siblings. A severely allergic child can find the problem compounded by being extra sensitive to a multitude of foods beyond the Big 8: mustard, chicken, or carrots, for example. So what else can a family do to better understand if a sibling who is asymptomatic today might develop food allergies tomorrow—or in the future? Traditionally, allergists do not perform testing before an individual has had an apparent adverse reaction to a particular food. The reason stems from the risk of finding sensitization to a food but not necessarily a formal allergy. So routine panel testing of foods is not recommended by the American Academy of Allergy, Asthma & Immunology or the American College of Allergy, Asthma & Immunology. The rate of asymptomatic sensitization to foods in the general population can be as high as 30 percent to 50 percent, yet these individuals are not truly allergic.

But if you already have a severely peanut-allergic child at home, and with all that's known and acknowledged about heredity, isn't there an increased risk for a peanut-allergic child to have a younger sibling with a peanut allergy? It's becoming more and more common that an allergy assessment by a qualified allergist of the younger sibling is a safe, prudent approach prior to the child's first anticipated exposure to peanut.

How about other allergies to, say, fish or eggs? If an older sibling is already having severe allergic reactions, shouldn't you inquire about younger children as well? Although it's not yet the standard of care to automatically have younger siblings tested, whether they are exhibiting allergic symptoms or not, it's wise to ask your healthcare provider about it. Families with a child who has a food allergy often wonder if a younger sibling should be screened before introducing potentially allergenic foods because the risk of food allergy in siblings of an affected child might only be minimally higher than in the general population. Or it might not. Further investigation could give you tremendous peace of mind if there is no issue at all, or at least more vital and necessary information moving forward.

Households with Multiple Allergic Children

When there are multiple allergies under one roof, having a mindful home with careful, special meal plans is essential. How to prevent food allergies from developing remains a mystery, but how to prevent an allergic reaction is clear: strict avoidance. In a household with multiple kids and multiple allergies, that isn't always easy. In some cases, parents decide to maintain completely allergy-free households, for example, going peanut-free when one or more children are severely allergic to peanuts. It may prove sensible in the home to just eliminate *all* of the allergens from the table instead of trying to juggle on various plates what brother can't eat but sister can eat.

If families find having the culprit food around causes too much anxiety for certain members, you can restrict all allergens. Some creative thinkers strive to become home kitchen Iron Chefs, coming up with innovative substitutions and delicious solutions that work for the entire family. That way, everyone can share the same meal at the dinner table and the person at the stove doesn't turn into a short-order cook. But it's important that each family determines its own comfort level—whatever works for your own unique family situation, structure, and desires.

Great Life Lessons for Nonallergic Siblings

One of the challenges of life with food allergies that is not talked about frequently enough is the emotional effect food allergies have on nonallergic siblings. All kids deserve to hear from parents what makes them unique, which is why it's so important to emphasize and nurture each sibling's unique strengths. Knowledge of that talent nurtures the child's self-esteem and sets him or her apart from siblings. Ideally, nurture a different strength for each sibling based on natural temperament and interests. Once you identify the talent, find opportunities to cultivate and validate it so each child can be acknowledged for his or her strength.

At the same time, don't talk yourself into senseless circles trying to always make things perfectly fair in your house—food allergy or not. Life just isn't fair. Instead, teach kids the skills that promote harmony so that they're more likely to cooperate. Of course, you can lend a sympathetic ear when your nonallergic child naturally complains from time to time about the situation and the lifestyle, but make it clear that it is not acceptable to complain directly to a food-allergic sibling. While siblings can be encouraged to settle their own disputes as much as possible, they will squabble regularly—but teasing and joking about food allergies and any aspect of the medical condition needs to be put in check right away. This is true even if it seems your allergic child can take the joke. Such behavior, if not checked, can lead your allergic child to harbor deep worries of inadequacy and internalize innermost negative feelings about his or her medical condition.

There's nothing worse than seeing a sibling in the throes of anaphylaxis—the fright and terror of the moment, the ambulance arriving, the subsequent hours or days in the hospital, and the return home to safety, protection, and love. So nonallergic siblings can easily be taught at a young age to be their brother's or sister's advocate, to provide a safe and stable environment where eating together doesn't feel exclusive. Teaching your nonallergic child ways to motivate his or her brother or sister to help with food allergy management can prove life changing. For example, he or she could remind the sibling to ask if a new food is safe before eating it. They can participate in role-play scenarios to help the sibling learn how to turn down food. A nonallergic sibling can develop lifelong confidence from the role of loyal protector. He or she can become a compassionate allergy superhero, as well, laser-spotting allergens. In camaraderie, he or she can share the same safe desserts so the sibling with allergies doesn't eat all alone and make sure that all the other kids know it. Many nonallergic children find themselves more compassionate later in life because it was needed from them at a young age.

Keep All Children Informed and Involved

Education is key. Food-allergic children and siblings must know that food allergies are serious. They must be knowledgeable about what is safe for each family member to eat, and they must be vigilant. They should know how to recognize signs of an allergic reaction and what to do. With practice, your allergic home can easily become your inner sanctum, a peaceful place of understanding where each member of the family is accepted as she or he is and is able to share hopes and even worries about this life-changing diagnosis and the management system required for survival within the safety of the family. What's needed to thrive in this world is a solid structure at home, where all of the children can practice skills and conversations so they are well equipped to handle the trials and tribulations and well-earned successes.

Part Three

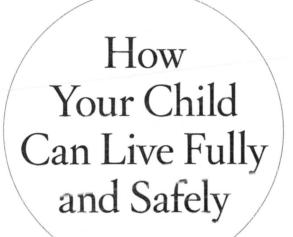

How Your Child Can Live Fully and Safely

8

Allergy Proofing
Your Kitchen
and Home

OUR HOMES should be our innermost sanctuary, a place to kick off our shoes and tune out the outside world as we dine and play and share time together. It's mercifully the one place we can pretty much guarantee we can stay safe from all of the outside food allergens in our dirty world and not have to fret and concern ourselves at the table about every muffin, every cookie, what might be hidden in the gravy. Organizing and maintaining an allergy-free home is certainly not an impossibility, although it takes some very specific, strategic planning and forethought to establish—and stick with—a solid game plan for safety and success.

The choice of whether to keep your entire residence allergen-free varies among families and will depend in part on the severity of your child's allergies, the age of your allergic children, and how responsible you can expect other members of the family to be. So brace yourself: Thoroughly allergy proofing the family home takes significant effort and time. But once you develop routines, implement housecleaning strategies, reduce allergens, and stick to a goal, you'll find your child—and the rest of you!— can breathe a relaxed, collective sigh of relief because an allergy-proofed home can be a vital part of your child's treatment program and help everyone in the home to stay relaxed.

Keep Your Landline Telephone

First of all, be sure you can reach out if there is an emergency. While a growing segment of society swears by only having mobile phones in their homes, a landline does have its benefits, especially in times of crisis. It may be worth it to have both, just so you know you're always covered.

Many households have disconnected their home phones and rely solely on cell service to stay in touch with the world. If you're thinking of joining the mobile-only movement, though, you might want to reconsider: Cell phones use a GPS-based method to report your location in a 911 emergency. With a cell phone, all calls must first be routed to the nearest emergency call center and then GPS is used to determine your location. That's fine when you're on the road, but if, for example, you live in a high-rise building, it won't indicate which floor you're on. A home phone is always connected to your address, including the apartment number, and so an emergency 911 operator knows exactly where to send help even if you can't talk.

Landlines still tend to beat out mobile devices when it comes to reliable connections and clear reception. And corded landlines that are connected to traditional copper will work when the power is out, which comes in handy when your cell phone can't be charged or isn't functioning. Many severe allergic reactions can occur within minutes of consumption, and a landline will always allow you to summon for help and assistance immediately—under any and all circumstances—if a severe reaction were to occur in your home.

Post Emergency Action Plans Around Your House

Post a list of allergens, emergency phone numbers, and procedures for managing an allergic reaction in the kitchen or pantry. Consistency is king here, and whether you have a relative helping to prepare dishes or a child care provider making the gang sandwiches, this is one more way to keep your home perimeter safe.

Stash Those EpiPens

You can add safety by storing a set of epinephrine auto-injectors in your kitchen—directly in the epicenter of all of the family food and meals.

Form a Safe Zone: Eradicating Hidden Allergens

Give your children a place to relax, where they can be safe and really, truly, enjoy their lives with all of their abundant and playful enthusiasm. Your home can be a safe zone.

Even with all the effort you put into keeping your home allergen-free, always listen to your body or your child's body, even if you haven't consumed and eaten something, because there can be allergens hidden in everything. If he or she exhibits any symptoms at all or you have a lingering doubt, it's always a good idea to call manufacturers or thoroughly check out their websites.

Throughout Your Home: Some paints and flooring contain food-allergic ingredients, but there are plenty of hypoallergenic choices in the marketplace now. When in doubt, check with the manufacturer. Only use a vacuum cleaner that has a HEPA (high-efficiency particulate arrestance) filter. Allergists recommend HEPA-filter vacuums because they reduce airborne allergens by trapping dust mites and other small particles and don't rerelease them into the air. This separates them from regular vacuum cleaners, which also take in dust, dirt, and allergic particles and allergens but unfortunately redistribute them right back into the air.

In the Living Room: This high-traffic area of your home, where guests and visitors congregate, is a useful place to serve as an allergy-free zone, a checkpoint for guests to ensure they haven't inadvertently brought in host gifts and snacks or are munching on allergenic treats themselves. This is particularly useful when there are many guests at once. Remember that food connects us all to each other because we all eat and so it is a universal activity and experience. Hence, this is also a good place to discuss allergies because explaining and discussing food allergies opens the door to understanding differences on a practical level.

In the Bathroom: Carefully check soaps, shampoos, and body lotions for allergenic ingredients. Don't forget the medicine cabinet: Some medications—even nonprescription, over-the-counter items that you have become used to keeping in your home—contain wheat, soy, and milk, so be certain to check both the active and inactive ingredient lists. Lipsticks and creamy makeup often contain wheat, nut oils, fish, soy, oh boy! Don't forget to pay special attention to your family's vitamin and supplement ingredients, too, as you may find them chock full of all sorts of "healthy" allergens.

In the Home Office: Many lick-and-stick adhesive stamps and envelopes contain wheat, and some older stationery set envelopes contain fish. If soy is to be avoided, you'll need to be extra careful with printer ink cartridges.

OUTSIDE CAREGIVERS IN YOUR HOME

Leaving your little one at home with a caregiver, especially when newly diagnosed, takes a special conversation and special trust. Communication is key, and every caregiver needs to have a comprehensive understanding of both allergen avoidance and how to respond in an allergy emergency. Set up a time to meet with your child care providers before they are scheduled to watch the children in your absence, and offer them compensation so they can spend some time shadowing you around your home, even for a full afternoon as a backup helper while they see how things roll in an allergen-free home and zone. Be sure to provide enough time for them to absorb information and to ask you lots of questions, and put everything down in writing together.

Make sure your caregivers understand clearly the house rules on what can and cannot be eaten around your child. Explain that takeout orders and any unauthorized snacks and treats are strictly off limits. However, you can ask your caregivers in advance if there are special foods and treats that they would like to eat (since, again, outside food is *not* a good idea) and purchase their favorites to stock in your pantry and refrigerator. Even something seemingly innocuous, like a granola/energy bar, can be made with peanut flour, for example; and a pastry or croissant to be munched on the go while kiddos eat their own lunch might well be glazed with egg wash.

(continued on next page)

(continued from previous page)

Keeping this kind of controlled environment within your home will keep you relaxed while you're away and provide your caregivers confidence to familiarize themselves with your new allergen-free lifestyle and to focus on a playful good time instead of food worries.

Nonetheless, even with a safe perimeter, all caregivers should be instructed on how to recognize the signs and symptoms of an allergic reaction—as well as how to use an epinephrine auto-injector. Post emergency contact numbers along with your cell phone number, and, if possible, the number of the location where you will be. Provide details on how and when to contact you, and include the phone numbers of others who may be able to help in the event of a reaction. If your allergic child has siblings, this is a particularly helpful area for a brother or sister to take charge and assist: They tend be excellent protectors and guards, and since they're so intimately familiar with the family, often they can easily spot allergens as well as subtle changes that could signal a reaction.

Many child care services offer caregivers who are CPR and First Aid Certified—which includes knowing how to use Epi-Pens. If your child care providers do not have this type of certification, show them how to use an epinephrine auto-injector and make sure they are comfortable using it. EpiPen training devices are the perfect way for everyone to familiarize themselves with what to do in case of emergency. Your child care providers must understand that once the epinephrine has been administered, your child must receive medical attention immediately—every single time. Caregivers need to know to call 911 even if it seems the symptoms have dissipated.

Guide to Kitchen Overhauls

When they receive a food allergy diagnosis, many families choose to do a complete cooking overhaul. Here are some tips for doing that.

Pots and Pans: You may decide to get rid of all of your old pots and pans and start fresh to eliminate any chance of cross-contamination and cross-contact from heated residual oils that cling to them. If you choose to do so, you can donate your old ones to a local Salvation Army or Goodwill. Cast-iron cookware is a mainstay in many kitchens; however, because it is often meant to be seasoned, particles from previous meals involving allergens can remain on the surface. The best and safest allergy-safe cookware is stainless-steel pans that are dishwasher safe, such as those from All-Clad, and cast-iron pans dedicated to only allergen-free food. Dishwasher-safe glass bakeware, like Pyrex or Anchor, is also excellent, as are stainless cooking utensils, silicone cooking utensils, and a special toaster dedicated for wheat-free and gluten-free bread, if needed.

Discarding All Unsafe Foods: An investigation through the refrigerator and freezer, pantry, and cabinets will yield a plethora of unsafe items. This is a great way to practice your skill at reading food labels, as you examine and discard items that clearly, or just might, contain the allergen. No family wants to be wasteful: Unopened items that have not passed their expiration date can be donated to a local food pantry or soup kitchen. These organizations don't accept items that are partially used or have been opened, but a neighbor or another family member outside the home might be happy to receive them.

Sanitation: Once you have removed allergenic items from the kitchen, it's time for your family to become a sanitization crew. You can use hot, soapy water. Or, as an extra precaution, you can use a solution of 1 tablespoon of unscented, liquid chlorine bleach in 1 gallon of water to sanitize your washed surfaces and utensils. Do not add more bleach than is recommended, and be sure to start off with a surface that has been washed and rinsed or the bleach will not be effective. Finish by allowing the area to air-dry. If you choose to dry surfaces with a towel, allow the bleach spray to remain on the surface for at least 30 seconds. Don't forget to wash cloths often using the hot cycle of your washing machine. Here are all the things you will need to sanitize:

- Cutting boards, plates, cups, and utensils will need to be run through the dishwasher at its strongest setting.
- Placemats, tablecloths, and oven mitts must be thoroughly cleaned and sanitized in a washing machine.
- Small rugs should be cleaned of food particles with soap, scrubbing, or in the washing machine.
- Kitchen and dining room chair cushions should be carefully vacuumed and washed.
- Clean the outsides of your oven and microwave, your fridge and freezer handles, and all of your kitchen cabinet pulls.

Sterilization: Food allergens can be transferred via unwashed hands or utensils, preparation surfaces, fryer vats, and even garnishes. One savvy chef taught me years ago to tell myself this sentence over and over: "I am not just allergic to fish, but I am also severely allergic to utensils that have touched fish." To sterilize utensils, use a sink, soapy water, and a clean dry towel. Fill a sink with soapy water, place utensils in the sink, and soak for 20 minutes. Then drain the sink and rinse your squeaky-clean utensils.

Now you have prepared an allergy-free kitchen, but since you have been used to cooking in your home without bearing allergies in mind, you will definitely need to relearn several aspects of meal preparations. This is especially critical when you are sharing your kitchen, say, for a Thanksgiving dinner with multiple chefs, bakers, and family cooks. Be sure to educate the whole family, and all visiting resident chefs, on your sanitation best practices.

You Are the Gatekeeper

There are ways your new kitchen needs to operate differently from before and from the ways that most household kitchens operate. Keeping track of them will help you communicate them to all who cook in your home, even if they are assisting you. You are the gatekeeper to your own kitchen, stocked refrigerator and pantry, and cooking processes in the home. Here are some habits that will help your home stay an allergen sanctuary.

Welcome to Cooking!

There's no getting around it: If your child has a food allergy, you will probably have to cook, at least sometimes. For some households, that's a snap. For others, if you've never cooked before or haven't done it regularly, the idea of learning to cook while dodging and darting around the food allergy can be daunting. Others love to cook but have never been in the situation of considering a multitude of necessary substitutions, which, in truth, can be intimidating for even a very experienced, seasoned home chef. Luckily, there are excellent resources that can help you find recipes you can use as is, adapt recipes for your own allergy needs, and track down unusual substitute ingredients. Chapter 11 offers a plethora of tasty substitutions and kid-friendly recipes for special events, but in the meantime, there's the nitty-gritty of daily meals in the family home.

Read Each Label Three Times

To keep allergens out, you'll need to become an avid label reader. Fortunately, packaged foods have ingredient labels that plainly state whether the product contains potential allergens. Law requires that the labels of foods containing the Big 8 food allergens (egg, milk, wheat, soy, fish, shellfish, peanuts, and tree nuts) note the allergen in plain language.

Take the extra step to read each label three times: first at the market, second before you place it into your fridge or pantry, and third right before you open it up to serve. This not only helps to catch an error on your end while busily shopping, but it is also a solid safeguard since manufacturers change their recipes from time to time and sometimes utilize new manufacturing facilities. In this manner, you have three fresh sets of eyes on each label—each and every time.

Make Yourself a Cheat Sheet

Make a list of all of the allergens. Keep it with you at all times. Include all alternative names or hidden sources of each allergen. This will be an important companion for grocery shopping. Then remember to check and recheck.

Prevent Cross-Contamination with Your Own Labels

Institute a labeling system for allergen-free foods. Carefully label each item and remind other family and household members of the dangers associated with cross-contamination.

Spend the Extra Time on Meal Planning

Family life can become admittedly hectic some days, and so whenever possible, try to prepare a menu before grocery shopping and make a list of all required items that you will need. Holidays and special milestone events take additional planning on top of the regular meals, so if any special ingredients will require a special trip to a certain store or need to be ordered by mail, allow adequate time to acquire them.

Prepare Speedy, At-the-Ready Meal Solutions

Keep plenty of simple and easy-to-prepare meals and snacks on hand—at the ready. This will prevent the last-minute frustration of "What can I make for a quick allergen-free meal?" Prepare large batches of freezer-friendly foods. Label each item carefully and include ingredients. This will allow for a quick meal for unexpected times when you may be unable to cook.

Perfect Cooking Methods to Avoid Cross-Contamination

A well-stocked kitchen isn't enough to safeguard your family from foods that could trigger an allergic reaction. You'll also need to study up on cross-contamination, which some refer to as *cross-contact*. Cross-contamination is the cooking or serving of different foods with the same utensils and surfaces and can occur when one food comes into contact with another food and their proteins mix, for example, on the same cutting board or the same serving utensil. As a result, the two foods blend in amounts so small that they can't be seen but each food then contains small amounts of the other food. Cross-contamination can happen at any time in the course of preparation. From a food's initial harvest in the fields, to setting it on a serving plate, cross-contamination, or cross-contact, is always a danger at any time for anyone with food allergies. In scientific terms, it is the transference of proteins. Sadly, *you can't cook off a protein,* so always remember: Cooking and heating the item does not reduce or eliminate the chances of a person with a food allergy having a reaction to the food eaten.

Make Washing Hands Absolutely Essential

Sanitize your hands thoroughly and often. Any part of the hands and arms that could potentially touch food needs to be washed. To wash your hands, first wet your hands and forearms with water. Next, add a dime-sized amount of soap. Use some "elbow grease" if you need to. Plain dish soap and water is best—there's no need to use an antibacterial soap. Soap is designed to lift dirt off surfaces with scrubbing, and warm water will help soap to work most effectively. There isn't any need to use excessively hot water; even cold water will work in a pinch. To get the hands clean, rub the soap over the surface of skin on the front and back of the hands, on the wrists, between the fingers, and just under the nails. It's the friction and rubbing, that agitating motion, that removes dirt from your hands. Lather with the soap for at least twenty seconds, away from the stream of water. Then rinse the soap away with warm, running water. Finally, dry your hands with a paper towel or a clean cloth towel. Never dry on pants or an apron.

Grocery Shopping and Sleuthing the Truth About Ingredients

Initial trips to the grocery store immediately following the diagnosis are all about becoming a food sleuth. A carefree shopping list and casual choices are now replaced with your ongoing action plan in your allergy-safe kitchen. Whether you have instituted a strict policy or will allow some allergenic foods into your kitchen, everything that enters has to be thought about in advance. Some families already read nutrition labels carefully for sugar and fat contents; now add to that a strategy to read food labels to ensure you are fully informed of allergens contained. FALCPA is an excellent amendment and is currently the best way to understand which packaged foods contain allergens. How do you read a food label? And what if it doesn't say anything about allergens—are those completely safe?

A company and its management may be subject to civil sanctions, criminal penalties, or both under the Federal Food, Drug, and Cosmetic Act if one of its packaged food products does not comply with the FALCPA labeling requirements. The Food and Drug Administration (FDA) may also request seizure of food products if their labels do not conform to FALCPA's requirements. In addition, the FDA is likely to request that a food product containing an undeclared allergen be recalled by the manufacturer or distributor.

Read for Hidden Allergens

First, read all product labels carefully, in their entirety, all the way through, before purchasing and serving or consuming any item.

Look for Bolded Statements

The next step to decipher a food label is to look at the ingredient list and check to see if the allergic item is listed in bold at the conclusion of the list. For example, "Contains: Soy, Egg." Okay, that's simple: If your child is allergic to soy and/or egg, you have received a warning and should not serve your child this product.

Notice Any "May Contain . . ." Statements

Look for a "May Contain" statement. You might see, "Contains: Soy, Egg. May Contain: Milk." Does that mean that if your child is allergic to milk, this product is okay to consume? Well, maybe, and this is where you will need to contact the manufacturer yourself, by calling or sending an email. The use of advisory labeling (i.e., precautionary statements such as "may contain," "processed in a facility that also processes," or "made on equipment with") is voluntary and optional for manufacturers. There are no laws governing or requiring these statements, so they may or may not indicate if a product contains a specific allergen. According to the FDA's guidance to the food industry on this issue, advisory labels "should not be used as a substitute for adhering to current good manufacturing practices and must be truthful and not misleading."

Call the Food Manufacturer

If you are unsure whether a product could be contaminated, call the manufacturer to ask about its ingredients and manufacturing practices. Keep in mind that you'll need to have the package of the product you're inquiring about with you when you call to verify safety; each bar code contains specific information, and some products are packaged in multiple facilities. The bar code tracks when and where each product is manufactured, so using an old package isn't safe; each time you will need to verify with the new package.

Manufacturing processes change from time to time, and especially during holidays production can increase dramatically to accommodate a multitude of extra orders. Products like chocolates, which may be made on dedicated allergy-safe equipment during most of the year, might suddenly be manufactured in mass quantities on many commercial lines. For food allergy safety, packaged products need to be checked each and every single time. You will definitely be surprised along the way and feel like an "allergy super-hero" when you catch something lifesaving on a food label.

Be Prepared to Alert the FDA

What about the recalls you see and read about in the news? Or what if you purchase a product that states it's allergy-safe and yet your child has an allergic reaction after consumption? Mistakes, unfortunately but realistically, are a reality of life. You should definitely help raise the flag by contacting the FDA. If you believe that the packaged product was mislabeled or contaminated, you can find an FDA consumer complaint center in your area and contact it by visiting this website: www.fda.gov/opacom/backgrounders/complain.html. You can also contact the FDA's Center for Food Safety and Applied Nutrition Adverse Event Reporting System by phone at (301) 436-2405 or by email at CAERS@cfsan.fda.gov.

Where to Find Safe, Allergy-Friendly Foods

As long as you are armed with the power to read labels, you will be able to find foods your child can eat. Here's a breakdown of the more common places to shop.

Internet Stores (WholeFoodsmarket.com, Walmart.com, Amazon.com)

Online retailers are available no matter your physical location and are an easy choice for a family's food allergy needs. In particular, online shopping tends to be easiest for nut allergies and celiac disease, since specialty online grocers exist for both of these conditions. These days, however, as vast as the Internet is, you can buy nearly any allergy-safe food online, including frozen or refrigerated foods. I utilize this option regularly, and it's a time and life saver for our food-allergic family. Even some foods I could find at the market are easier for me to order in bulk online.

The only two drawbacks to online shopping are shipping costs—sometimes coupons for free shipping are available—and the need to plan ahead since you will need to anticipate ordering nonallergenic foods in advance of when you want and need them.

Food delivery boxes are available in most major cities, ranging from organic fruits and vegetables to a complete list of items and a recipe to make a meal swiftly yourself. One example for peanut and tree nut allergy is a new online food delivery box called Pnotbox (www.Pnotbox.com), available with a monthly subscription. It is shipped to your front door chock full of allergy-safe granola bars, cookies, crackers, and a rotating variety of snack treats. With food allergy needs now well recognized in the mainstream marketplace, and with some website surfing of your own at home or on your smartphone, there are plenty of similar options that can be arranged.

Specialty Supermarkets (Whole Foods, Trader Joe's, and Fresh Organics)

Specialty supermarkets are also sensible and viable options for allergy-safe grocery shopping. These stores generally offer a variety of products for a number of restricted diets, and some even offer coupons or pamphlets detailing which items in their stores are free from the Big 8 common allergens. Specialty supermarkets also often offer their own high-quality store brands of common allergy-safe alternatives, usually found right next to the brand-name competitor, except theirs are more cost-effective.

Again, here is where contacting manufacturers to learn of their "May Contain" best practices is useful. Once I placed a telephone call regarding a specialty supermarket brand of organic ketchup, already certain there was no chance of the product containing nuts. Guess what? It did contain nuts and was prepared on a shared line with their specialty brand peanut butter. These calls to verify can sometimes yield a surprise answer, and with good practice making the calls—which only takes a few minutes—you can keep your family that much safer and protected from an allergic or anaphylactic reaction.

Chain Supermarkets (Safeway, Vons, Lucky)

Like snowflakes, no two chain stores are exactly alike. Supermarkets vary by neighborhood, and even by region and season, in the amount of allergy-safe food they stock. As a general rule, these foods are shelved in the "Natural Foods" or "Health Foods" section in larger grocery stores. You will definitely be able to locate dairy-free milks, especially soy and rice, at all supermarkets. You're also likely to find large selections of wheat-free foods, especially breads, which are usually in the frozen aisle. There are also cereals and pastas to accommodate kids on gluten-free diets, plus some nut-free cereals and lunchbox-friendly sandwich spreads like SunButter. Most chains place the sunflower butter or alternative toasted soy WOWBUTTER options smack in the midst of the allergenic peanut and nut butters.

Warehouse Clubs (Costco and Sam's)

The great aspect of shopping at warehouse clubs is how cost-effective they are for the family budget. It's always wise to factor in whether you are going to have to drive out of your way to get to the warehouse club or if it's located near places where you already travel on a routine basis. These establishments are able to keep prices low due to the no-frills format of the stores. They have definitely adapted to the times and are improving, but many may not offer plentiful allergy-safe options. Still, with some poking around and a keen eye on the mailers they send out regularly, some of your family's allergy-safe grocery needs can likely be met, with dairy-free milk boxes and some nut-free snacks. The bulk prices tend to make this option worth a little extra work, and with so much variety and square footage, who knows—you might just find a new favorite allergy-safe treat along the giant aisles, like our family has.

9

Eating
on the Go

OUR YOUNG CHILDREN soak up everything we do like little sponges and observe us closely—and naturally mimic food cues from us, their parents. Establishing calm, stress-free mealtimes for food-allergic children sets them up for a future where mealtimes are associated with a comfortable, social experience. It's important to prepare your food-allergic child to avoid anxiety around food as they mature. Food is an integral part of our lives: from the ritual of preparing, to the social dynamic of breaking bread together, to the communal cleanup postmeal. Incorporate your little one into each aspect of how to share meals so he or she can carry this forward into a young adult life. Your food-allergic child will be able to go out on social occasions, and eventually even on dates, more relaxed and able to focus on friends at the table instead of being consumed with food worries.

Lunchbox Items

It all starts with that little lunchbox when you send your child out into the world. A lunchbox is a good beginning for reinforcing the comfort and safety of managing your child's food allergy. It's the special way children know they are being loved and cared for when they're away from your family table. No doubt children feel confidence and protection when they sit down among friends and open up their lunch containers to eat communally with peers and share that social time. There are recipes in chapter 14 that might help you pack your child's lunchbox.

Cafeteria Foods and Buffets

Steer clear of this style of meal preparation and service. Multiple platters and bowls, with utensils that can get jumbled and placed into other foods, are a formula for disaster. You might get lucky and avoid a reaction, but the odds are that with so many hands and so many various dishes and so many allergens comingled into the buffet style of dining, it's only a matter of time before there is an accident and a reaction. Food for allergic individuals is best prepared with no chances for cross-contact, in dedicated serving bowls with dedicated utensils, in its own area rather than in close proximity to allergens.

Allergy-Friendly Restaurants

The app AllergyEats is a great way to find restaurants that have been vetted by the allergy community. While our various allergies and their severity may differ, one fact all us allergic families can agree on is that once we discover a safe haven and a dining spot at which we can safely eat, we become veritable regulars at the establishments. Better yet, we're often able to establish highly personal relationships with the managers and staff so that when we arrive, it can almost feel like a home away from home—an extra-nice treat for a family with food allergies. Establishing your favorite haunts is always fun, but be prepared for disappointments along the way as a chef ventures to a new restaurant, your beloved general manager is suddenly gone, or there is a menu overhaul—seasonal or otherwise. It's necessary to check the menu each and every time, always at the ready to ask questions.

Tips for Ordering

Calm, clear, and direct communication is essential. Keeping control of your food allergies at a restaurant can be intimidating, especially when the kitchen is behind closed doors; however, learning how to eat out safely with food allergies is absolutely vital for your social experience. But here is where communication is key because information needs to travel all the way from the front of the house back to the busy chefs. It's important to make restaurants aware of your food allergy, even if you dine there regularly. It's unrealistic to expect them to remember your medical condition when they don't manage it in the daily way you do. Explain your condition thoroughly before any food is brought to the table and request that certain ingredients not be used in your food. I always check with the waitstaff and chef to ensure that fish is not cooked in the same skillet or in the same oil as other food items. It's also good to make sure that your dishes are not prepared with the same utensils or on the same work surfaces as your allergen, or you will be subject to cross-contamination.

How to Talk to Waitstaff

When your family's life depends on it, ensuring you are having the same conversation with a busy waitperson who is handling multiple special requests at any given moment is critical. Your child's life may depend on it. The good news is that the food and hospitality industry as a whole has risen to the challenges us food-allergic diners have presented to them. Waitstaff certainly don't seem surprised when we discuss food allergies at our tables with them. The key is to ensure the information is explained clearly and that both you and your servers check in frequently with each other when ordering, after the order is placed, and when the food arrives at your table.

It's very important to not apply undue pressure to the waiters, demanding they adhere to your food-allergic needs. It is better, I find, to be flexible and allow them to say "no" if they are not sure they can accommodate your family medical condition. A scenario in which a stressed-out waiter, aiming to please, overpromises because you are too demanding can have dire consequences. So always make sure to allow them the freedom and comfort to tell you that they simply can't guarantee a safe meal. There are plenty of restaurants where an allergy action plan is in place behind the scenes in the kitchen, and if one is not, you are wise to avoid the establishment altogether. An open relationship with the waitstaff, a keen understanding of what it can and can't promise, and a meal built on a foundation of excellent communication and vigilance creates a forum for successful experiences dining out together.

Fast Food Can Be Safe Food

We have at last reached an era and a climate where "fast food" has largely and mostly been replaced with "good food, quickly." This is especially helpful for people with food allergies, since much attention is being paid to nutritional information and the quality of ingredients used. Everyone from the cashier up to management is well versed on useful food information. The conversation overall seems to have evolved so that everyone is speaking the same language regarding oils used, cross-contamination, and even whether genetically modified foods are incorporated into on-the-go meals. There's a newfound sensitivity and thoughtfulness regarding food allergies when dining on the fly, and a few fast-food joints pride themselves in particular on nut-free dining: Krispy Kreme Doughnuts has no nuts, ever, and In-N-Out Burger is also a nut allergy champion. There is not a nut or cross-contamination on either menu, anywhere. The larger franchises, such as McDonald's and Wendy's, keep allergen and nutritional information up to date on their websites. While there is some maneuvering necessary at the big fast-food eateries, there is a welcome awareness and a keen eye maintained by the corporations, reflected in new menu layouts that are available online.

A Snacking Strategy

Gone are the days when you could grab any little snack you desired for your child out and about in your adventures. The reality now is that even the littlest munchies—even just one single tiny bite—need to be carefully thought through to keep your kiddo safe from allergic reactions. Trace amounts of an allergen can still produce a life-threatening anaphylactic response. Children are hungry and growing and in need of easy and on-the-go nutrients. I still remember my own daughter's intense disappointment when the ice cream truck would come jangling up to the playground in the summer—an environment rife with allergenic nuts. Eventually, I found these to be teachable moments: Ice cream, while delicious and certainly to be enjoyed from time to time, isn't a nutritional necessity. Instead, of course, we could plan ahead a little, and with minimal forethought even bring to the playground our own little cooler with a safe frozen ice cream snack.

Do Your Research and Plan Ahead

The act of spontaneous eating is something food-allergic individuals have to live without and become accustomed to, sadly. It's just a matter of fact. Better to learn about the best nutritional choices, and safe ones at that, to prepare your son or daughter for a lifetime of healthy decisions. These in turn can give them a much longer life, food allergies or not.

10

Safe and Happy Holidays

FROM EARLIEST CHILDHOOD, food represents family, community, and belonging. Social life, vital to our emotional and psychological health, almost always revolves around food at the holidays, and our celebrations invariably involve sharing the appropriate food for the occasion. Holidays bring cheer and abundant festive eating. Most of our friends and family are fortunate enough to not have to consider a relationship with food the same way we do; instead, when they are hungry, they just eat anything at all. When they attend celebrations, they expect and receive food and enjoy it without worry. Whether you are a host or a guest, it's pivotal to try to understand each other's position about food so we can learn and grow and teach each other together.

Holidays are plentiful and always around the corner, with typically very food-centric components incorporated into these celebrations. Food allergens lurk in many traditional Thanksgiving, Hanukkah, Christmas, Kwanzaa, and Easter dishes. There are ways to celebrate with all of the traditional festivities and trimmings, both at home and visiting.

Offer to Host

The easiest way to keep these holiday parties their very safest is to host your own, if feasible. This way, you know exactly what's being prepared and how it is being prepared—of course.

Educate Your Guests Beforehand

Holiday gatherings are perfect opportunities to remind family and friends about your child's allergies. Speak up before the crowd arrives for all the fun, and remind everyone that cross-contamination and cross-contact of food allergens can happen easily. A minuscule amount of an allergy protein may be invisible to the eye, but it's enough to trigger an allergic reaction for someone with a food allergy. Remind guests in the invitation that you have an allergen-free home and offer suggested alternative and substitute holiday gifts. Just be sure that everyone attending your holiday parties is reminded or told about your child's food restrictions. Remind yourself that guests won't always remember your child's food allergies—despite multiple conversations, sometimes—and that they are excited about the holidays and can be distracted. If you recall that certain folks just don't seem to remember, it's okay to double-check with them before they bring a cornucopia of holiday food and gifts into your home.

Remind Your Child to Stay Safe

Remind your allergic child to avoid food sharing, even at home, during the holiday event and to ask you—every time—before eating any food that you haven't prepared yourselves. Also instruct your child to practice especially good hand hygiene, washing them frequently.

Limit Dishes People Bring

Many people want to be helpful and share in holiday traditions by bringing a bounty of something homemade and they don't realize that even a small amount of an offending food—crumbled on top of a main dish, as a festive garnish, for example—could cause a serious reaction. They need to steer clear of foods with a likelihood of cross-contamination: Food items purchased from bulk bins, deli cases, and salad bars aren't typically sanitized and are subject to whatever was in the various containers beforehand. If they want to bring something, you could politely suggest that they bring something safe—perhaps a holiday beverage of some kind, or a bottle of wine that goes nicely with the meal, or holiday-themed napkins or decorations. Holidays are traditionally a time of sharing, and guests like to feel included in the celebrations. They have a natural inclination to share seasonal gifts with you and your family. If someone calls you with little notice on his or her way over and insists on picking up a last-minute, quick something or other to contribute, you could suggest that he or she can safely contribute bagged ice, safe factory-sealed beverages, fresh flowers for the holiday table, or board games and art projects.

Ask for Ingredient Lists

For potlucks, buffets, or well-meaning contributions to your table, ask guests to provide ingredient lists. If an item is store-bought, ask them to bring the wrappers with the label. If guests write up ingredient cards to place in front of their dishes, the food-allergic child can easily identify what's in each dish, you can be comfortable and certain of what your child is eating, and you can locate the cook if you need more information about how the dish was prepared.

Use Creative Substitutions for Traditional Dishes

You are the master chef in your own allergy-safe home, and you don't have to forego traditional dishes: As needed, you can swap in whole-grain, gluten-free flours for wheat, ground flaxseeds or applesauce in place of eggs, and tried-and-true (and tasty) sunflower butter in place of peanut butter. These are all easy swaps that will yield similar results, but here's a tip: It's best to taste test all of the substitute recipes before serving them to guests. Definitely do a trial run, as things like cooking times and textures may need to be adjusted.

Stay Calm and Immediately Remove Allergens That Arrive

If allergenic holiday items accidentally sneak their way into your home, stay calm, cool, and collected; stash them away in a safe place; and donate them to a neighbor or another relative at the end of your holiday event. If the item is dangerous in any way, or if you or your child is uncomfortable, take it out of your home immediately and throw it away, far from your child's reach, into a lidded and secure trash container. A public garbage can on your street corner keeps it out of reach, out of sight, and out of mind. When you return home, thoroughly wash and sanitize your hands. Then get right back to enjoying your holiday party without worry.

Encourage Guests to Express the Holiday Spirit in Creative Ways

The sign of a good host is how welcome the guests feel in the home, and with a little creativity, everyone will feel equally received and appreciated during these wonderful times of the year.

Suggest items they can bring to share in the holiday spirit: games, art supplies, crafting gifts, holiday-themed napkins, balloons or paper decorations, picture frames, fresh flowers, potted plants. A holiday guest brought my family wacky holiday-themed sunglasses one year to create a slapstick and silly, allergen-free mood. It was such a great gag gift that no one even thought about food allergies for the entire duration of the party. For once it was a nontopic. Feel free to let your creative side shine through for your host and promote a less food-centric celebration. Your food-allergic friends and family will be grateful!

Being a Guest and Staying Safe

If you have plenty of time for advance planning for an event, you can work out many of these details with a positive and proactive action plan by contacting the host—with notice—to ask about the holiday catering and what foods will be safe. It's useful to keep in mind that during the holidays busy hosts and hostesses are often working behind the scenes to accommodate more than one guest's distinctive needs, so focus on the end goal and stay courteous (even if you feel you are reminding for the millionth time—maybe it's only the first time you have someone's full attention). It's easy for people who don't live with food allergies to forget about how harrowing it can be for us and our children, so repeat yourself even if you know you've said it all before and they are not remembering.

Contact Caterers Beforehand

You can offer to unburden your host by offering to place a call or send an email to the caterer yourself, since the chef will know more about the food than anyone else and you know more about the allergy than your host. Expert, meet expert! Chefs are well versed in food accommodations and substitutions, ranging from allergies and sensitivities to diabetes, mercury levels, Kosher, low-carb, vegetarian, you name it. Most caterers and cooks are remarkably savvy, and some are trained specifically in health and integrative nutrition practices. They know how to have a conversation with you that can yield a positive outcome for everyone, especially your busy host. Upon arrival, you can arrange to check in personally and meet up with the chef you have been speaking with to confirm your child can safely eat those certain items discussed free from cross-contamination and cross-contact. Chefs are generally warm, accommodating, and extremely knowledgeable about various food needs at special events—they are in the business of food, after all.

Come Prepared with Snacks and Desserts

If you're headed out to a friend's or a family member's home for the holidays—or even a restaurant or hotel banquet hall—and if you're not sure that there will be completely allergen-safe food, your child can always have a snack or light meal beforehand so that he or she doesn't run the risk of going hungry. Or you can stash something on the go in your pocket; an allergen-safe energy bar is portable and nutritious, so if your child becomes hungry at the celebration, there's something readily available—yet completely safe—for a quick munch. You can also pack snacks such as fresh fruit with sunflower butter packets, carrot sticks with hummus, air-popped popcorn, or your own homemade trail mix with cereal, seeds, and safe chocolate chips. For easy festive desserts, melt chocolate chips as a dip for dried apricots or allergen-free cookies, or bake apples sprinkled with cinnamon and brown sugar and top them with allergen-free whipped topping. Bring them with you tucked into a coat pocket or purse.

Be Aware of the Environment

Upon arrival at your holiday destination, do a quick scan of the room to identify hazards. If your child is severely allergic to nuts, for example, you can ask your host to put any bowls of nuts or candy containing nuts away for the evening and briefly explain why.

Be on the alert for goody bags or party bags and always ask what's inside. Piñatas, for example, might contain baubles and trinkets and toys, but they may also include edibles—it's best to check in and politely inquire. We each have our own family traditions that we celebrate with great gusto during our holidays, so we understand that hidden allergens may very well pop up, but we are equally well prepared to ask the right questions, without judgment, in order for the celebration to be equally wonderful for one and all.

Sit Next to Your Child

Depending on your child's age, you may choose to have him or her seated beside you during the holiday meal. This will ensure that you will be alert if those eating nearby accidentally spill or share unsafe foods and you are poised to keep unsafe foods out of reach of young children with allergies.

Offer to Bring a Dish

If your holiday event isn't catered, then perhaps it's groups of friends and family cooking. If your event is buffet style, you can offer to bring your own food, a safe entrée in your own serving dish, with your own utensils. This allergy-safe dish can be placed to the side or separately in the kitchen so that there are no mistakes and cross-contamination or cross-contact with your serving utensils. Additionally, you can offer to work with the host to create a safe menu. Often a food can be made safe simply by slightly adjusting the recipe. If the Martha Stewart gene hasn't skipped you, try suggesting that you can prepare the food alongside your host as an assistant chef and to help with label reading and preventing cross-contamination or cross-contact.

Desserts Can Be Worrisome

Desserts typically can be laden with allergens, many hidden, and with so many homemade holiday desserts on a table, there are usually no labels to verify ingredient lists. Wisely, some families choose to avoid these holiday dessert buffets completely and instead participate in a postparty, separate "second" dessert on the way home at a safe bakery. Or they plan ahead and dine on something festive prepared back at home after the main holiday celebration. When baking at home for the holidays, finding allergy-free substitutes is a big part of celebrating milestones with food allergies. Initially you'll probably find that one thing that seems to work really well, but then when you use that substitution in another recipe, you may find that it doesn't work as well. It's really all about trial and error. Once you discover foods that can be substituted for those that your child is allergic to, you can start cooking and baking recipes that you've always loved again; many recipes are ahead in chapter 14. You'll probably discover new holiday favorites as well.

Holiday Gift Suggestions

Of course, relatives and friends will want to give your child gifts for the holidays. There are increasingly plentiful options now for holiday-themed gift baskets for people with food allergies. It's also easy to suggest nonfood options, such as books, toys, or gift certificates. Here are some great resources.

Divvies.com prepares and ships stylish vegan gift baskets that are full of treats that contain no nuts, peanuts, egg, or dairy. They specialize in gourmet cookies, chocolate, and popcorn.

Vermont Nut Free Chocolates has something for every holiday occasion, and they offer a wide variety of allergy-friendly gift baskets produced entirely in a dedicated nut-free facility.

Build-A-Bear Workshop now has a loveable, adorable velvet puppy that is certified asthma friendly and free of allergens. There are many allergenic teddy bear options now. Because many children with food allergies also have asthma, and some plush animals may be stuffed with nut shells or soy-based fibers, certified allergy- and asthma-friendly stuffed animals take the worry out of gift giving and provide your relatives with options to still splurge on your family.

Books make terrific gifts. If you have an avid reader in your home, children's books about food allergies also make great gifts at any time of the year. However, if you are buying for a child with soy allergies, attention should be paid to avoid board books printed with soy-based inks.

The Halloween Switch Witch

Probably the trickiest holiday for children with food allergies is ever-spooktacular Halloween. Traditionally, every October 31, children dress up in costumes to engage in trick or treating; they might also decorate and carve jack-o'-lanterns, visit haunted attractions, dunk and bob for apples, and watch scary movies. So while there are popular activities aplenty, typically this holiday primarily comes down to two main themes, the double *c*'s: costumes and candy (candy, candy).

Traipsing from door to door asking for candy that is allergenic and that your child can't eat can easily dampen the festive mood on Halloween eve. How can all of this tradition be converted into more useful treats for children with food allergies? Naturally, these kids can easily feel left out. Enter the Switch Witch, who lives on a little island along the dark side of the moon in Hallow Heights and simply adores candy. Of course, all witches love candy, but none as much as her, and she has the biggest candy stash of all the witches. She loves candy so much that she's even willing to trade all her favorite toys to little boys and girls in exchange for their candy stash. Of course, the boys and girls can keep a little bit of candy for themselves, but the more they give the Switch Witch, the better their toy will be.

The Switch Witch flies from building to building on her broom with her black cat on the back, and they fly in through the window with magic (it does not need to be open). She takes all of the candy the child leaves out and puts it into a sack, and then she takes out a shiny black bag that is full of toys and books. She leaves one toy or book for the child to thank him or her for the candy. Then she leaves just as quickly as she came, on her broom, out to visit other children and perform more switches. By early morning, she returns home to Hallow Heights, where she sorts the candy into large glass jars. That night, all of the other witches come to visit, and the Switch Witch doles out the candy they want. They eat their candy with her, share stories of Halloween, hear about what toys she brought to the children, and come back night after night for a treat.

You know how most pictures of witches are flying near the moon? That's because they are on their way to Hallow Heights to visit the Switch Witch and share in her gigantic candy stash. She devours the children's candy over the course of the entire year. And just as she runs out, luckily it's Halloween again and time for another visit.

If the notion of a witch sneaking into your child's room is too scary, she could go by another different name. Some families call her the Candy Fairy (cousin, perhaps, of the Tooth Fairy?). The end result is the same: a festive and joyous Halloween night experience with "Switchcrafting" to make the food allergies an integral component of the magic.

11

Family Getaways

YES, YOUR FAMILY can venture out on a road trip, a camping trip, even a summer abroad if the adventurous spirit moves you. Traveling with your food-allergic child and family can naturally stir up all sorts of anxious feelings. You may be worried about being far from home and having access to the foods and treatments you need. One way to ease your anxiety is to prepare yourself for all kinds of situations that may come up on your trip. Talk to others who have traveled to the area or, if possible, locals who understand the culture and traditions and can tell you what to expect. If someone else is doing the planning, make an appointment to sit down and discuss your child's needs and provide detailed written instructions for the trip. And remember, you know the best way to manage your child's food allergies. What you do at home will often work on vacation, too. So it's absolutely possible to get away and enjoy it all with advance planning and some strategic prep work.

Plan Ahead

Instead of trying to push worries aside, use them as a guide to prepare yourself for the kinds of situations you might face in a new place. Remind yourself that your anxiety is real and understandable. Not only do you and your family have to stay safe in a new place, but you might also have to handle any social concerns that arise, like asking for special accommodations, avoiding certain activities or places, or explaining the need to prepare and eat your own safe food and meals. You already know how to manage your child's food allergies; you do it all day, every day. Those same strategies that help you cope at home can work well on trips, too.

Medications: Don't plan to rely on local pharmacies for your prescriptions because medications may not be the same overseas. Instead, plan to take all of your child's meds with you. Discuss travel plans ahead of time with your pediatrician and allergist to be sure you have all the medicines you need for your child, from antihistamines and inhalers to epinephrine auto-injectors. If your insurance company or pharmacy tells you that it limits how much of a prescription you can fill at once, a letter from your child's doctor explaining the situation may allow an exception to the policy.

Emergency Plans: Ask your doctor to write and sign a food allergy emergency action plan for your child and keep it handy. It's best to also research local area hospitals and doctors ahead of time online. Make a list on a three-by-five index card, keep local emergency numbers on you at all times during your family vacation, and find out where local emergency medical help is and how long it will take you to get there from your hotel, vacation rental, or campsite.

Insurance Coverage: Make some phone calls to find out in advance if your insurance will cover the costs of overseas or out-of-state medical care. If not, it may be prudent to invest in travel insurance for your trip.

Packing Medications: Pack your epinephrine auto-injectors and antihistamines in your hand luggage so that they're easily available, and be careful to wrap and pack your child's emergency medications carefully so that they don't get crushed or leak.

Rules About Medications on Airplanes

Transportation Security Administration (TSA) guidelines state that as long as your medication is in its original packaging and is clearly labeled, you shouldn't have issues bringing it on an airplane. If you're concerned about carrying your child's auto-injector onto your flight, ask your doctor for another note explaining what the medication is for specifically and why you need to be carrying it to prevent potential confusion or delays at security checkpoints. The TSA is an agency of the U.S. Department of Homeland Security, which has authority over the security of the traveling public in the United States. According to the TSA blog (http://blog.tsa.gov/), you can bring your medication in pill or solid form in unlimited amounts as long as it is screened.

- Medication in liquid form is allowed in carry-on bags in excess of 3.4 ounces in reasonable quantities for the flight. It is not necessary to place medically required liquids in a zip-top bag. However, you must tell the officer that you have medically necessary liquids at the start of the screening checkpoint process. Medically required liquids will be subjected to additional screening that could include being asked to open the container.

- You can travel with your medication in both carry-on and checked baggage. It's highly recommended you place these items in your carry-on in the event that you need immediate access.

- TSA does not require passengers to have medications in prescription bottles, but states have individual laws regarding the labeling of prescription medication with which passengers need to comply.

- Medication is usually screened by X-ray; however, if a passenger does not want a medication X-rayed, he or she may ask for an inspection instead. This request must be made before any items are sent through the X-ray tunnel.

Ensuring a Safe Plane Ride

Not surprisingly, some airlines are more accommodating than others when it comes to food allergies. When you are considering a family vacation, it's useful to understand the various policies and accommodations. You will be sealed up in a metal tube for hours and hours, with food-y recirculated air aplenty, far from the emergency room, after all. So plan ahead and call to discuss your needs to determine which airline is the right choice for your family well before you make your reservations. If you're not feeling 100 percent confident that your family will be safe, don't travel with that airline.

Food Onboard

You can request a safe snack, but it's a good idea to bring your own allergy-safe food along onboard—just in case. Depending on the airline, some might offer gluten-free or allergy-friendly meals. If you do order a special meal when booking your tickets, you may want to call a day or two in advance to verify that it will be available on your flight. Whichever airline you select, it's okay to bring your own food with you on a flight—even on an international flight. As long as you don't pack any liquids or gels over three ounces, you won't have issues with airport security. You can bring homemade meals, safe packaged foods, even fresh fruit and vegetables to snack on during your flight. But remember that customs usually prohibits bringing fresh produce into foreign countries, so you'll likely need to finish eating your fruits and veggies during the flight or be prepared to toss them in the trash afterward.

Alternatives to Hand Washing

Washing hands frequently and keeping them away from your mouth, nose, and eyes is generally a great way to avoid accidentally coming into contact with allergens, but when traveling you can't count on having access to copious amounts of soap and running water. So on an airplane, a good supply of hand wipes ensures that you can clean your hands and wipe around seating areas where contact with allergens is highly likely.

MISCELLANEOUS TIPS

► Upon check-in, ask if you can board your flight early so that you can have the opportunity to wipe down your seating area without delaying other travelers.

- When you board, remind the flight crew of your family medical condition.

- Unless your child is traveling solo, he or she doesn't really require the additional "I Have a Food Allergy" sticker since you will all be together in the small space with the bracelet donned. But if he or she is traveling solo, you can make this sticker out of a simple name tag.

- Even if you have taken all the proper health steps, travel emergencies can happen, and enlisting the help of those around you can help you take responsibility for your own safety. So don't hesitate to inform the people sitting around you.

- You may also decide to carry a medical release form on board, signed by your child's doctor, which would authorize others to give your child epinephrine.

Book a Hotel Room with a Kitchen

One of the cornerstones to eating safely with food allergies is being able to prepare your own meals. Check ahead, but most hotel and motel rooms are equipped with minirefrigerators, and at the very least this will make storing safe foods from the supermarket or leftovers that don't require cooking easier. Many hotels have business-class rooms available, which contain a small kitchenette with a stovetop or a full kitchen. Just ask—often when you mention your child's medical condition, you will receive a free upgrade. When traveling on a budget, hostels and guesthouses will include a shared kitchen space. In a community kitchen, your vacation box with all of your own cooking utensils will be necessary. Even *your own sponge* is a must-have: Small particles and pieces of allergenic foods become caught in a shared sponge and cross-contaminate your dishes, even if your prepared meal is totally safe.

Pack a Vacation Kitchen Box

It can be reassuring to bring your kitchen on vacation right along with your entire gang. There's no need to leave it behind! This box is your key piece of luggage: You are now traveling and bringing your own kitchen from home along with you. You can check this as you would luggage and unpack it on the other end of your adventurous travel. Or you can mail it to your destination.

Before you depart, get yourself two sturdy moving boxes from a local shipping store or from U-Haul. Keep one folded and pack it early with your clothing and essentials, and then load up the second box as you would a moving box: bubble wrap, moving tissue, the works. Now pack your supplies, depending on your family's needs. You can include things like

- Containers for storage and leftovers
- Cookie sheet
- Cups, plates, and cutlery
- Cutting board
- Foods that fulfill your essential needs
- Ice tray
- Measuring cups and spoons
- Napkins
- Pizza pan
- Pots and pans with their lids
- Salad spinner
- Toaster

A trip to a local grocery store completes this box. As you pack to return home, if your first box is well worn from usage, it's time to put your unused second box to use and repack your safe supplies. Have the pristine second vacation box shipped directly from your hotel lobby back home or find a local post office—it will be there shortly after you arrive back home.

Planning Where to Eat Ahead of Time

The best way to boost confidence and calm nerves is to research and plan your trip thoroughly. It also helps to talk through any worries with supportive friends and family who will be joining you on your vacation. Not only can they help you avoid risky situations, but they can also be your emotional support system.

Save yourself time trying to figure out where you and your family should dine once you reach your destination, and ameliorate danger by organizing this part of family travel well in advance. If you want to plan ahead, you could even call grocery stores and ask about certain brands or ask them to place a special order or hold items for you. Upon arrival, buy your basics and favorite safe foods; return back to your hotel, rental home, or campsite with all your necessities; and get cooking with the family.

Right now, only Massachusetts and Rhode Island have passed bills mandating food allergy awareness programs in restaurants. Both states require restaurants to display posters about food allergies and designate employees to undergo allergen training. In 2012, Maryland's legislature passed a bill requiring restaurants to display a food allergy awareness poster and creating a task force to study the issue. Nonetheless, certain restaurants have become hardwired to make safe and delicious allergy substitutions, and the "fast-casual" dining segment has moved particularly aggressively toward accommodating allergies.

Use your time wisely, beforehand, by finding out what allergens are in the local cuisines so that you can judge where it's safe to eat out during your vacation. You can surf the Internet and check online to find out where your destination city has restaurants ready and willing to accommodate your food allergies.

Then confirm your child's allergies while making your reservations and again at the table. Don't just ask if a menu item includes your child's allergy trigger. Instead, be more specific and ask to speak to the manager or chef who will prepare the food so that you can find out what's in it and how it's made. Some restaurants provide special menus for dietary restrictions, and many kitchens have matrices of dishes on the menu noting what allergens they contain.

Keep in mind, however, that you are a long way from home and your familiar pediatrician and allergist. Just because a hotel or restaurant claims it can handle food allergies doesn't mean it can actually keep your child safe. So it's particularly important to carry your child's rescue medications to a new restaurant. Don't hesitate to have a conversation with your waiter and, ideally, your chef about your meal so that you can discuss your child's food allergies and potential sources of cross-contamination before you order.

Another tip: Use a free online web mapping service, like Google, to book your restaurant reservation as close as possible to a local market or grocery store, if possible, so that if it's not feasible or safe for your child to eat there, you can dart out to buy something else quickly to bring back to the table, with the restaurant's permission.

Learn to Talk About Allergies
in the Local Language

When you check the Internet, you will no doubt notice that there are a lot of websites that offer translations of allergen information into a variety of different languages. Allergy translation cards indicate your family allergy needs in the language and dialect of the region you'll be traveling in. Some of these sites will send you laminated cards in the mail for a small fee, while others offer free translations for you to print out yourself from your home printer to make international travel easier.

If you're ordering a translation card or set that needs to be delivered, be sure to order early enough to check for completeness. Checking for accuracy is key. Make certain your translation cards explain all of your dietary needs and mention the possibility of cross-contamination, ideally recommending that completely clean utensils, pans, and cutting boards be used for your food in the native language.

Consider laminating cards you print yourself for durability or backing them with cardstock. If you're going abroad and already speak the language, then you have an advantage: Talk directly to the grocery store, restaurant, and hotel managers. If, however, language is a barrier or if your family just needs more answers, you can plan ahead and seek help from food allergy organizations, travel agents, trip coordinators, or local friends and relatives. Think on it and prepare a lengthy list of questions before making your calls and then take careful notes.

If you have your allergy translation cards at a restaurant, even if you have made a reservation in advance and spoken to the waiter, you should still request that your card be passed along to the chefs prior to your meal so that they can assess exactly how your child's food should be safely prepared. Keep in mind that different cultures have different understandings about their own food, and so you may find you need to specify—in great detail—which allergic foods your child can't eat. For example, with my fish allergy, I might also state that I can't eat chowders, ceviche, sushi, or California rolls, even though that means reeling off a list instead of just saying "fish." If anything looks questionable or if the restaurant doesn't seem to fully understand, then we stick with options we know are safe or we choose to find another restaurant.

Summer Sleep-Away Camps

There's a new bumper crop of camps that have arisen nationwide to meet the needs of severely food-allergic children. Some are day camps and some are sleep-away camps, but this new strain shares one trait in common: They strive to provide a completely worry-free experience where young people with food allergies can build confidence and independence and enjoy a summer rite of passage away from their parents without the threat of their allergens on the premises. Food awareness is the focus at these camps, and they don't serve the top Big 8 allergens. Some allergy-free camps are also sesame-free and gluten-free to accommodate almost every food-allergic lifestyle.

The real world certainly isn't allergy-free, however, and some parents might prefer a more practical environment where older tweens and teens can learn to manage and coexist in an allergy-filled world. Gaining the skill to communicate effectively while advocating for oneself is a useful tool in all aspects of life. Depending on the camp's administration, medical care, and emergency protocols, it can be possible and enriching to attend a regular sleep-away camp with friends and siblings. In choosing a camp for my nut-allergic daughter, this is our annual personal choice.

It's essential to prepare ahead of time. Camp staff, physicians, parents, and the campers themselves need to work together to minimize risks. As a parent or guardian, there's plenty you can do to arm yourself with knowledge about your youngster's traditional summer camp. Some questions to ask include the following:

- Is the camp accredited?
- Does the camp have designated personnel to handle an emergency?
- Does the camp have a policy for managing food allergies?
- Most importantly, do camp counselors know how to inject epinephrine?
- Where exactly will medications to treat an allergic reaction be kept?
- Will ingredients be labeled in the campers' dining area?
- What about safe snacks in cabins?
- Are the food service personnel educated about creating a safe meal free of cross-contamination?
- If the camp is in a rural area, how far away is the closest emergency facility and does it have a doctor available 24/7?
- How will the camp communicate your child's food allergy information to counselors and activity leaders?
- Will campers be outside the camp on field trips (boating, biking, or hiking), and if so, where will medication be kept in this scenario?
- What about allergen avoidance during arts and crafts, such as egg cartons, paints, or bird feeders?

If you're unsure the kitchen staff will comply, your camper may want to provide his or her own coolers of safe snacks and even meals, complete with dedicated, safe cooking utensils. Make sure the area where these are stored will be designated as "allergy-free" to avoid any and all cross-contamination.

Camp counselors and activity leaders can be key in the line of defense, so ensure that they are fully aware and trained. Some camps have tours in the late spring months so you can get a hands-on understanding of the facility, but if not, if you provide the camp with advance notice, you can arrive with your camper early and tour the facilities, speak with staff, and get comfortable. It's absolutely possible to survive and thrive with food allergies at summer camp.

Part Four

Ways You Can Protect Your Child

12

The ABCs
of School Rules

ONCE YOU HAVE CAREFULLY constructed a protective strategy and action plan around your food-allergic child to prevent food exposures at home, and to a lesser extent at the homes of family and friends, it's time to face the realities of his or her days at school. You've followed all of the techniques, allergy-proofed your home, become an allergen-free party planner, checked every pet food label—you have a system in place that works. When it's time for your little one to leave the nest and go off to school, it can feel like entering a minefield, as allergenic dangers seemingly lurk *everywhere* all at once.

In an organized, well-ventilated cafeteria, your child can steer clear of the peanut butter and jelly sandwiches that pop out of lunchboxes. But what about the surprises, like the constant stream of food trickling into the classrooms for snacks, parties, and rewards? How about the booby traps hidden in crafts like papier maché planets or peanut butter bird feeders? Because young children first attending elementary school have had less overall exposure to potential allergens, they are at greater risk of having their first reaction: twenty-five percent of anaphylaxis reactions in schools occur among students without a previous food allergy diagnosis, when it is discovered in the school setting for the first time.

The severity of a food allergy differs with each person. Sometimes allergy moms and dads are called "hysterical" and "overreacting" when we are neither. Annoying, sometimes downright insulting generalizations like these are tossed around, and we serve our children best when we just let them slide off our backs like Teflon. So take a deep breath and once again become your child's advocate.

Gather Allies Among School Staff

The most significant factor in how schools and districts measure up to keep our allergic children safe is that personal, human touch: the presence of an informed parent (probably you), nurse, teacher, or other staff member who serves as a champion for food allergy awareness and preparation. Who your allies will be depends on how your public school district works or what resources your private school offers.

Inquire About School Nurses

In a public, unified school district, school nurses are deployed differently: Some work part-time at several schools, and others are full-time nurses devoted to one school. If your school only has a part-time nurse, there may be less overall awareness about allergy precautions and fewer staff members who are trained to administer epinephrine injections in an emergency. You will need to ramp up your efforts to educate teachers and recruit awareness allies.

If you are fortunate enough to have a nurse devoted to the children at your school, make the best possible use of him or her as an extension of your own diligence. Ask the nurse to help you and your child's teacher come up with strategies for tricky situations that are unique to the school, the particular classroom, or your child's specific allergy. And be sure to go over the emergency response plan.

Teachers Become the Gatekeepers

Share with your child's teacher that you have a mutual goal: to create a safe environment that still allows for maximal growth and development of each and every food-allergic child. Longtime high school teacher Sophie Abitbol, a fifteen-year veteran educator in Burlingame, California, shares that she's had anaphylactic teens in her class with gluten and dairy allergies. Sophie acknowledges that she keeps an extra eye on them and has been careful to keep their allergies in mind when she brings in food for the class, as she is familiar with several of the news stories with terrible outcomes. Sophie has a balanced outlook and explains that her pupils "are old enough to manage what they need to do" but notices that her allergic students need some reminding from the school nurse.

There May Be Policies That Assist You

Despite differences between schools and districts, fortunately state policies and resources have created some uniformities in the past several years. For example, most school districts are required to have policies to accommodate children with food allergies, and at some schools specific "safe" cafeteria tables are set aside for students with food allergies. There are also strict rules about sanitation procedures and hand-washing guidelines for students.

Give Your School the Basic Medical Facts

Whenever school starts for the year, be sure that the new teacher, nurse, or administrator has the six facts that give educators at your child's school the medical knowledge they need to confidently care for food-allergic kids. Here is what they need to know:

- A food allergy is an overreaction of the immune system that can affect any system of the body, including the respiratory, cardiovascular, gastrointestinal, and skin systems.

- Ingestion of even a minute amount of the allergen can trigger this overreaction and cause a variety of symptoms, ranging from mild nausea or itching to anaphylaxis (a systemic allergic reaction that can kill within minutes).

- There is no cure for food allergies. Strict avoidance of the allergenic food is the only way to prevent a potentially life-threatening reaction.

- An allergic reaction can occur up to two hours (and sometimes, although rarely, up to four hours) after ingestion.

- The severity and progression of an allergic reaction is unpredictable: a seemingly mild reaction can turn fatal within minutes.

- Anaphylactic reactions are treated by prompt administration of epinephrine. Time is of the essence and may mean the difference between life and death. An immediate call to 911 and then transport to an emergency room must follow. A second repeat dosage and administration of injected epinephrine may be required.

Sharing How to Avoid the Allergens at School

Because strict avoidance of the allergen is the only way to prevent reactions, it is critical that teachers and staff be given practical information on how to make the classroom, lunchroom, playground, and field trips safe for food-allergic students. You can help teachers and staff who supervise your food-allergic students with yearly, end-of-summer, or beginning-of-school-year check-in meetings.

Demonstrate How to Read Food Ingredient Labels

Meet with your child's teacher and bring sample food labels with you so that you can go over what he or she needs to be on the alert for. Make copies of your own personal cheat sheets that have all of the names used for your child's allergen and give them to the teacher. Don't be afraid to impress upon the teacher how important it is to read labels three times: when the food or craft material is bought, when it is brought into the classroom, and before it is given to your child.

Go Over All the Ways to Prevent Cross-Contamination

Don't rely on district policy to ensure that proper sanitation and cleaning methods happen. When you bring up methods that prevent cross-contamination, such as hand washing, surface washing, and the like, you are emphasizing just how important this is. Teachers may be inspired to go the extra mile to keep your child safe.

Alert Them to Sources of Hidden Allergens

It is vital to remind teachers that the food we eat is not the only potential source of allergens: They need to check art supplies—like clay, paints, and egg cartons—as well as hand lotions, soaps, and anything else you are aware of that contains your child's allergen.

Tell Them Your Child's Symptoms of a Reaction

You know the observable symptoms of your child's allergic reactions, so share what teachers need to watch out for. Also share the ways your child communicates these symptoms to be sure that they know when your child is telling them something is wrong.

Make Sure They Are Ready to Apply Emergency Procedures

While we hope that this will be clear as a bell, it's better to be safe than sorry. Ask them to review what they will do if a reaction occurs.

Establish a Communication Pathway

Let the teacher know how he or she can best alert you to issues that might affect your child's food allergies, such as upcoming field trips or parties, projects, dynamics between children, your child's self-care, or anything that might come up in the course of lessons. Showing your engagement will encourage them to reach out to resolve challenges more readily.

GIVE THEM THIS BASIC CHECKLIST

✓ Notify all substitute teachers and teacher aides about students' food allergies.

✓ Avoid using food in lesson plans, such as math lessons and art projects.

✓ Don't use food as an incentive or reward.

✓ Minimize the use of food in class parties or celebrations.

✓ Consider food allergies when planning for field trips, and be sure to include parents and the school nurse early in the planning process.

✓ If the classroom has a pet, check the ingredient labels on the pet's food.

Make an Allergy Emergency Kit for Your Child's School

Allergy emergency kits are a necessity for your family's survival strategy and especially useful for children with food allergies who spend time away from home at school. Make sure whoever will use the kits at school knows and understands the signs of food allergy reactions and anaphylaxis. Store these items in a durable case, clearly marked—ours is fire-engine red. Here are the supplies you will need to include:

✓ Injectable epinephrine (EpiPen), along with written instructions for administering it

✓ Oral antihistamines, such as Benadryl

✓ Fast-acting asthma medication and spacer, if applicable and prescribed

✓ A durable card (laminated, if possible) with the name and phone number of your child's physician, the hospital you prefer your child be taken to, contact information for family members, and insurance information

✓ Any other items your child's allergist has recommended you keep handy in case of severe reaction.

Update the kit regularly. At least once a year, check each of your emergency kits to be sure that none of the medications have expired and replace as necessary. Also, make sure the insurance and emergency contact information on your card is current.

The Stock Epinephrine Bill

When a third-grade student in Tennessee who had been stung by a wasp developed welts on his neck and had trouble breathing, fortunately his school nurse had the necessary dose of epinephrine to counter the allergic reaction. A law Tennessee enacted in 2013 makes it easier for schools to stock the lifesaving drug. The nurse said the emergency room doctor told the boy's parents that he probably wouldn't have survived without the injection. There is currently a bill under consideration in the legislature that will lead to additional potential safeguards for children with allergies. Bill 1171, also called the Stock Epinephrine Bill, would allow schools to keep epinephrine auto-injectors on hand for trained staff to use on students experiencing anaphylaxis—even if they don't have their own prescription. It also provides legal protection for staff members who administer it. Check with your state to see if it has passed laws allowing—or even requiring—schools to have epinephrine on hand.

The idea is to allow teachers or other school staff to immediately curb a life-threatening reaction during the crucial minutes before paramedics arrive. The measure would mainly protect students who have undiagnosed allergies that are triggered at school for the first time.

Making Accommodations Clear with 504 Plans

Children with food allergies are entitled to have a 504 Plan in place at their school that provides children with disabilities accommodations to fully participate in school. A major provision of the Rehabilitation Act of 1973 (29 U.S.C. § 794) requires school districts to provide all students, regardless of disability, with a "free appropriate public education." This provision, found in Section 504, applies to any condition—physical, mental, or emotional—that might interfere with a student's ability to receive an education in a public school classroom, subject to external review. As a result of the Americans with Disabilities Act Amendments Act of 2008, students with severe food allergies are also increasingly getting 504 Plans.

As part of the plans, the students' parents, physician, and often the school nurse make a list of accommodations, which may range from using extra sanitizer at the students' lunch spots to allowing them to be first through the cafeteria line to ensure their food is prepared and wrapped first. Having this plan in place provides an excellent framework for us to discuss self-care responsibilities with our children and for us parents to clearly discuss with school staff what their children can and cannot do for themselves with respect to keeping safe from allergens in a school setting.

Some do question going to all the trouble of creating a 504 Plan when you could just sit down with your child's teacher and principal before the school year starts and come to an informal agreement. The major difference between a 504 Plan and this sort of casual discussion with teachers and administrators is that a 504 Plan is a recognized, legal document. So if the plan is not enforced, parents have legal recourse to the U.S. Office for Civil Rights or to the local courts, depending on the jurisdiction. (An attorney is your best source of answers for specific legal questions about your 504.)

If your child's school is reluctant and resistant to making changes that you feel are necessary for your child's food allergy safety, going through the outside evaluation process and getting a 504 Plan may be the best way to protect your child in the classroom. Even if your relationship with your school has been cordial, having a formal, legally enforceable plan may prevent your relationship with the school from becoming adversarial because expectations for all parties—parents, children, classmates, food services workers, nurses, and administration—should be clear after the 504 is completed.

Not all students with food allergies are eligible for a 504 Plan, so you should check with your state. Ultimately, 504 Plans are completely optional, but many, many states do have them already in place. To be considered eligible for a 504 Plan, a student must have a condition that "substantially limits one or more major life activities," which are then defined further within the law. The school district evaluates students to determine eligibility prior to creating the 504 Plan (if students are denied 504 Plan protection, parents have the option to appeal the ruling). The factors that the school district considers in evaluating the student include the severity of the condition and the student's ability to provide self-care. Thus, a kindergarten student with an anaphylactic peanut allergy who cannot yet read would almost certainly be considered eligible under the terms of the law; a high school student of typical intelligence with a milk allergy whose major symptom is rhinitis (a runny nose) likely would not.

Managing Field Trips

Extracurricular activities and field trips are wonderful, team-building opportunities for your child to interact with classmates outside of the school setting and offer unique learning opportunities while engaging students on a higher level and making learning fun. The school field trip has a long history in American public education. For decades, students have piled into yellow buses to visit a variety of cultural institutions, including art, natural history, and science museums, as well as theaters, zoos, and historical sites. These adventures can be safe and enjoyable with clear communication and careful, advanced detailed planning. Here are some things to work out with a teacher or group leader beforehand:

Create a Food Allergy Action Plan: Discuss this as early as possible in trip planning to allow for timely adjustments to be made. Students with food allergies should turn in a Food Allergy Action Plan to the group leader. This can be done by carefully reviewing the itinerary and meal locations and considering possible hidden allergens.

Encourage school nurse to attend trip: A nurse can be an invaluable resource on a school trip where students have food allergies.

Offer to co-chaperone the trip: Depending on the age of your child and the severity of the allergy, you can request to attend the trip to ensure safety.

Review emergency response protocol: Review student food allergies and the corresponding action plan with all of the trip chaperones. Identify the students with food allergies, discuss what foods to avoid, explain corresponding allergic reaction symptoms, and review the Food Allergy Action Plan.

Ask that all snacks with allergens be banned: Request this in case it is not already being done. Parents can be informed of food allergies at a pre-trip meeting or with a note sent home with ample notice. Teachers can confirm with each student before they board the bus that they have not packed foods containing the allergens. Students with allergies can be encouraged to pack their own safe food to eat while traveling and given a pre–field trip reminder to carefully read food labels before packing the meals.

Check expiration dates and always have medicine and auto-injector close by: Ask teachers to confirm medicine is not expired before departing for the trip. In addition to the student carrying his or her medications, ask teachers or chaperones to carry the food-allergic student's medications with them in a small bag, clearly labeled, wherever your child goes. In the case of a severe allergic reaction, quick access to medications can make a lifesaving difference. Keep all staff and chaperones informed about who will be carrying the student's medications.

Check cell phones and cell phone chargers: Ensure that the teachers or leaders have cell phones that are charged and available to call for help in an emergency. This is a good chance to remind them to always call 911 if epinephrine is administered.

Update emergency contact information: Confirm that this information is correct so that you can be notified immediately if something happens.

Prepare Your Child for Safety—and for Fun!

Have a conversation with your child, gently reminding about the importance of not sharing food and to remember his or her other food allergy strategies but, most importantly, to experience all that the trip has to offer him or her. Because now that everyone has done their homework and planned accordingly, you can confidently focus on reminding your child to enjoy the field trip and take notice of the wonderful learning opportunities at hand.

13

Birthday Parties
and Group Celebrations

IT'S CRITICAL for our children to socialize with one another and
to prepare to be immersed in environments with all sorts of
different other individuals, and group celebrations are an integral part of this dynamic. What kid doesn't love a birthday
party? While tons of fun, birthday parties can be the least con-
trollable experience for the food-allergic family. There will be
people you don't know and who don't know your child; lots of
food incoming from different sources, much without food labels; and events that may take place at a home, event center, or
park that is unfamiliar.

Educate Everyone You Can

As vigilant and supportive as we are at home in our own walls,
it does take a village to support our food-allergic children, and
our villagers have an especially important supporting role: to

help keep our kids safe from their potentially life-threatening allergic reactions. The unglamorous reality is that each birthday party at school or for your son's or daughter's friends is a potential minefield that could conclude with a harrowing trip to the emergency room. Forty percent of children with a food allergy have already experienced a severe or life-threatening allergic reaction. I cringe to think that some other parents, those who have children without food allergies, probably (hopefully) only a few, may dismiss our issue as someone else's problem, a burden, or an annoyance.

Some of them must ruminate, "Isn't it hard enough to meet our own kids' needs without worrying about someone else's?" In this context, they may view restrictions on their food options to accommodate our kids with allergies—in their strong opinion—as an infringement on their rights: "Why should we be inconvenienced by nut-free play spaces, daycares, or schools just because someone else's child has an allergy?" Sometimes the best defense is a strong offense, and if you sense a reluctance from another parent, pause for just a moment to gather your inner strength and do your best to sensibly try to explain your lifestyle. Often it helps to describe and share your child's most recent allergic reaction so there can be a concrete cause-and-effect understanding. There are some times, however, when people are not open or interested in hearing about our family food allergies, nor in accommodating them. Sometimes it's best to walk away, whether that is to keep your child safe or to preserve a relationship. This does not make the other person a bad person, although it may suggest that he or she is not an ally in food allergy support.

It can make the situation a difficult one for managing food allergies. If you have to attend an event hosted by one of these individuals, make your own best choices to keep the drama out of it and keep your child safe. Inversely, what someone says may not be an accurate communication of their intent. A host may intend to help or be inclusive without knowing the best way to do so. Usually people have the best of intentions, but without clear communication both can leave the party feeling misunderstood. In general, people do not intend to be disrespectful, hurtful, or unsafe about food allergies, and most party hosts genuinely want everyone to have positive experiences. Clear communication about expectations and sharing your education about food allergies can empower both the food-allergic family and your friends and extended family.

And, sometimes, the most stubborn parents from the outset will surprise you and become your biggest allies—once they have spent time with your family and can see your food allergy life through their own eyes up close. Building a dialogue and creating an ongoing conversation is key, and while it can be slightly uncomfortable to take the reins and open up a discussion with a parent you don't know too well from your child's classroom, it's really the only way to make this medical condition more personal.

Throwing Your Own Birthday Bash

When you are throwing your own allergy-free party or celebration, with a little planning and creativity, it's feasible and manageable to keep allergens at bay. The most effective way to do this is to shift the focus away from food. At many birthday parties, food-allergic children who attend as guests are unable to eat most of the usual goodies and are, unfortunately, often resigned to passing on that cookie or yummy-looking cupcake.

So, for your own event, opt to not make food the focal point of the party. Instead, plan a fun theme such as a carnival, pool party, or skating party where the children will be busy playing games or having fun exercising rather than eating. Play pin the tail on the donkey or do an art project rather than hitting a piñata filled with candy, and provide nonfood prizes for games and goody bags. Here are some more things to consider and tips for navigating them:

TIPS FOR YOUR PARTY

- **Party bags and favors:** Double-check at your party supply store to ensure any edibles are allergen-safe.
- **Party venue:** Bowling alleys and even pools sometimes have common food and beverage areas. Be certain to contact any rental facility well in advance to make sure it's able to safely accommodate your allergic child. When you find one, discuss your family's food allergy with the manager and devise a plan to meet your safety needs.
- **Party piñata:** Either check all prepared piñata candy prizes yourself or purchase an empty piñata that you can stuff with allergy-free candies and treats.
- **Snacks and cakes:** If you are ordering snacks and cakes from a bakery, be certain to explain the food allergy medical condition thoroughly. With a little planning, the birthday celebrant can eat everything at his or her own party.
- **Guests and gifts:** Let guests know in advance, in writing or on an electronic invitation, that gifts for the birthday boy or girl must be allergen-safe.
- **Inclusion:** Do your best not to make the allergic child feel special or different, but instead create group and community activities that allow him or her to join in and be one of the gang.

Visiting Others' Birthday Parties

Food allergies when attending birthday parties outside your own home can feel scary for both the host and guests, but there are a lot of ways to party without stress, worry, and (it's okay to admit) even resentments. Everyone is together to celebrate—and with practice, you can subtly do your part to keep that in the forefront. Like most parents, I don't wish for my child to feel different in social settings, but I also don't want our dietary differences to be an unmanageable chore for our host. That means I'm willing to do whatever I can on my end to make the process easy and even will go the extra effort—wherever that leads. Fair or not, sometimes life for an allergic family is like that, and we parents have to do what it takes to keep our children safe and emotionally and socially healthy.

Preparing the Host

Empathetic hosts are the key to unlocking this vital social experience for our children. I ask them if they are familiar with food allergies in general, and then I get more specific. Most importantly, I remind myself that the host may have heard from other parents regarding other special accommodations, so I stay mentally fit if they are distracted or initially don't seem to understand why I am calling them and making such a big deal. I hang in there, take a deep breath, and gently try to get on the same page with them, all the while remembering that they may possess zero frame of reference for my family's food allergy lifestyle and can't fathom the dire need for this perhaps seemingly annoying conversation.

Be Ready for What Will Be Served

Ask the hosts what exactly, *specifically*, will be served at the birthday party. If they haven't planned that part yet or are simply too busy to know the menu at that time, I ask politely if they wouldn't mind keeping the empty packages with the food labeling once they go shopping so that I can investigate the wrappers myself upon arrival—if that's helpful for them.

Offer to Stay at the Party

Remember, upon arrival, if you sense that your hosts are not comfortable being responsible for your child, you can always offer to stay at the party with your child. Don't force the responsibility on them. They might be grateful for your presence if you can also help with managing the activities. Gradually, the other parents will start to feel more confident about caring for your child. Give them time. It takes patience for everyone to understand each other's medical needs, particularly when we are not used to managing them on a day-to-day basis.

TIPS FOR BEING A GUEST

- **Bring your own food:** If it helps your child, "match" your food—bring a cupcake if the host is serving cupcakes. These decoys can be enjoyed safely with the rest of the gang.
- **Watch out for guests bringing food:** The host may not be aware that these extra goodies are incoming.
- **Do not accept food for your child without checking ingredients:** Many people are not aware that food additives can be derived from common allergens. Be careful with homemade items that may be cross-contaminated.

- **Bring sanitizing wipes:** Bring plenty in case they're needed to clean surfaces (spoiler alert: They usually are).
- **Remind your child about the rules:** Until you're sure your child is in charge of his or her allergy, always remind him or her about food allergy safety rules before attending a friend's party. These include not eating anything without clearing it through Mom or Dad and never sharing food from another guest's plate, no matter how tempting.
- **Alert others with a tag:** For very young children, you can purchase or make "I Have a Food Allergy" stickers or even order food allergy tattoos online for your child to wear at the event.
- **Keep medicines near:** Always have your child's up-to-date epinephrine auto-injector and other medications on hand at group celebration events.

There is a unique balance we have to strike as parents of food-allergic children, particularly if the allergy is severe. On the one hand, you must make sure your child is kept safe, but on the other, you want to allow him or her to fully participate in and enjoy all life has to offer. Social activities are important for your child's happiness and self-esteem, and going that extra mile creates a lot of happiness for our kids when they can enjoy a "normal" birthday party experience right alongside the gang.

14

Allergy-Friendly
Recipes

AFTER YOUR CHILD is diagnosed with a food allergy, it's a scary, seat-of-yours-pants time. However, there's absolutely no need to put away all of your favorite cookbooks or to pass by every recipe you come across that contains allergens. As helpful as recipes written for allergies are, it's a tremendously useful skill to be able to adapt your own favorite family recipes or those you find in cookbooks and magazines.

This will come relatively easily to experienced cooks, but the learning curve can be steep for any parent who is new to the kitchen. We're all busy, and favorite family meals can be modified in even the busiest household.

Here is a cornucopia of my family's favorites on these pages, all tried and true, from our own kitchen. Getting inventive with alternatives and substitutions can have mixed results at first, but the outcome gets better and better with practice, and soon enough new traditional dishes are revamped with their own special flair and touches. Some of our best "mistakes" in the kitchen have yielded the tastiest allergy-safe plates, so experiment, experiment, experiment.

Discovering safe seasonings and spice blends also enhances family mealtimes, and with a phone call or visit to a website you can be assured of which spices and brands are best for your family's allergic needs. There's never a boring meal when we creatively season something—in most cases it can change the nature of the dish completely. Allergies really, truly don't need to place a limit on the flavor profile of our menus. Even if store-bought spice blends aren't safe for your gang, there are always fresh herbs that can be purchased or grown in tiny pots in a kitchen window to add depth of flavor and a pop of color so the feast is as appealing as it is delicious.

For Your Wheat-Free Kid

Having a wheat allergy (or gluten sensitivity or intolerance or even celiac disease) is no reason to miss out on big flavor. Here are some substitutes for wheat in recipes:

- For breads, rolls, muffins, brownies, and other baked goods, substitute barley flour if your allergy is to wheat and not gluten. It performs the best of the alternative flours because it's one of the few grains, besides wheat, that contributes some gluten. Some stores also sell gluten-free baking flour. It can be used for making everything from cakes and cookies to breads and muffins.

- Substitute wheat-free pasta for noodles called for in recipes. Made from a variety of grains, including quinoa, corn, potato, rice, and beans, wheat-free pastas are widely available in stores.

- Eliminate breadcrumbs in recipes like casseroles, fried chicken, eggplant parmesan, or meat loaf and use shredded parmesan, crumbled wheat-free crackers, or cornmeal (depending on the recipe).

- For sauces and gravies, thicken the mixture with cornstarch, potato starch, or tapioca starch.

- For sauces, gravies, or creamy dressing, thicken and blend the mixture with pureed soft or silken tofu.

- For pancakes and waffles, use flour from other grains such as oat flour, rice, or barley.

Whether you start with homemade bread or choose a simple, colorful, Cuban-inspired bean and rice salad (use gluten-free distilled white vinegar and toss in some shredded chicken for even more protein) or even wheat-free vanilla cupcakes, some of these recipes are destined to become lunchbox staples.

WHEAT-FREE SESAME SANDWICH BREAD

Prep Time: 1½ hours

Cook Time: 45 minutes

3 tablespoons unsalted butter

4 tablespoons sesame seeds

½ teaspoon unflavored powdered gelatin, from 1 (¼-ounce)
   envelope

1 teaspoon sugar

2¼ teaspoons active dry yeast, from 1 (¼-ounce) package

3 large eggs, room temperature

¼ cup buttermilk, room temperature

1 tablespoon molasses

½ cup tapioca flour

6 tablespoons chickpea flour

¼ cup almond flour

¼ cup coconut flour

¼ cup amaranth seed flour

¼ cup sorghum flour

2 tablespoons yellow cornmeal

2 tablespoons potato flour

2 tablespoons cornstarch

1½ teaspoons xanthan gum (a thickening agent, easy to find
   at Whole Foods or Trader Joe's)

¾ teaspoon kosher salt

Position rack in middle of oven and preheat to 425°F.

Butter an 8-inch x 3¾-inch x 2⅜-inch loaf pan.

In small saucepan over moderate heat, heat butter until hot but not
smoking. Stir in 3 tablespoons sesame seeds and sauté until seeds
are golden brown and fragrant, about 4 minutes. Transfer mixture to
small bowl and let cool to room temperature.

In small bowl, sprinkle gelatin over 2 tablespoons cold water. Stir,
then let stand until softened, about 5 minutes.

In large bowl, stir together sugar and Ð cup warm water (105°F to 115°F). Sprinkle yeast over and let stand until foamy, about 5 minutes. Add 2 eggs, buttermilk, molasses, butter–sesame seed mixture, and gelatin mixture, and whisk to combine.

In large bowl of electric mixer fitted with paddle attachment, whisk together tapioca flour, chickpea flour, almond flour, coconut flour, amaranth flour, sorghum flour, cornmeal, potato flour, cornstarch, xanthan gum, and salt. Add wet ingredients and beat at moderate speed until dough is aerated and holds its shape, about 4 minutes. Scrape down bowl, then beat at high speed for 1 minute. Transfer dough to prepared pan and smooth top with rubber spatula. (If helpful, use a wet hand to smooth completely.) Cover loosely with plastic wrap and let rise in warm place until dough is just level with top of pan, about 1 hour.

In small bowl, whisk together remaining egg and 1 teaspoon water. When dough has risen, lightly brush egg wash over top, then sprinkle with remaining 1 tablespoon sesame seeds.

Bake bread until firm, about 30 minutes, then carefully turn loaf out of pan and continue baking directly on oven rack until bottom sounds hollow when tapped, about 15 minutes more.

Transfer to wire rack and cool at least 1½ hours before slicing.

Store bread, wrapped in aluminum foil, 3 days at room temperature, 1 week refrigerated, or 1 month frozen.

Yields: 10 lunchbox sandwiches

WHEAT-FREE BLACK BEAN & RICE SALAD

Prep Time: 10 minutes
Cook Time: 40 minutes

1 cup long-grain Jasmine brown rice
¼ cup extra-virgin olive oil
1 Italian frying pepper (mildly sweet flavor) and cut in ⅓-inch cubes
1 medium red onion, finely chopped
3 garlic cloves, smashed, peeled, and minced
2 cups freshly cut super sweet corn kernels (from two ears)
1 teaspoon kosher salt
1 15-ounce can black beans, rinsed well and drained
1 tablespoon distilled white vinegar
Freshly ground black pepper

Bring a medium saucepan of salted water to a boil. Add the rice and cook, stirring occasionally, until just tender, about 25 minutes. Drain and rinse well with cold water until cool. Transfer to a large bowl.

Heat 2 tablespoons of the oil in the same saucepan over medium heat until hot. Add the frying pepper, onion, and garlic and stir until slightly softened, about 3 minutes. Add the corn and salt and cook, stirring, until just heated through, about 1 minute. Transfer the vegetables to the bowl with the rice and toss to mix.

Add the beans, the remaining 2 tablespoons oil, and the vinegar and toss well. Season with plenty of pepper and toss again.

Yields: 6 cups

ALLERGY-FRIENDLY VANILLA CUPCAKES

Wheat-free, Egg-free, Dairy-free, & Peanut-free, too!
Prep Time: 15 minutes
Cook Time: 22 minutes

2 cups garbanzo–fava bean flour
1 cup potato starch
½ cup arrowroot
1 tablespoon plus 1½ teaspoons baking powder
½ teaspoon baking soda
1 teaspoon xanthan gum
2 teaspoons salt
⅔ cup coconut oil
1⅓ cups agave nectar
¾ cup unsweetened applesauce
3 tablespoons pure vanilla extract
grated zest of 1 lemon
1 cup hot water
Allergy-friendly vanilla frosting (recipe to follow)

Preheat the oven to 325°F. Line two standard 12-cup muffin tins with paper liners.

In a medium bowl, whisk together the flour, potato starch, arrowroot, baking powder, baking soda, xanthan gum, and salt. Add the oil, agave nectar, applesauce, vanilla, and lemon zest to the dry ingredients and combine. Stir in the hot water and mix until the batter is smooth.

Pour ⅓ cup batter into each prepared cup, almost filling it. Bake the cupcakes on the center rack for 22 minutes, rotating the tins 180 degrees after 15 minutes. The finished cupcakes will be golden brown and will bounce back when pressure is applied gently to the center.

Let the cupcakes stand in the tins for 20 minutes; then transfer them to a wire rack and cool completely. Using a frosting knife, gently spread desired amount of vanilla frosting over each cupcake. Store the cup-cakes in an airtight container in the refrigerator for up to 3 days.

Yields: 24 cupcakes

ALLERGY-FRIENDLY
VANILLA CUPCAKE FROSTING

Wheat-free, Egg-free, Dairy-free, & Peanut-free, too!
Prep Time: 6 hours (includes chilling time)
Cook Time: 10 minutes

1½ cups unsweetened soy milk
¾ cup dry soy milk powder
1 tablespoon coconut flour
¼ cup agave nectar
1 tablespoon pure vanilla extract
1½ cups coconut oil
2 tablespoons fresh lemon juice

In a blender or a food processor, combine the soy milk, soy powder, coconut flour, agave nectar, and vanilla. Blend the ingredients for 2 minutes.

With the machine running, slowly add the oil and the lemon juice, alternating between the two until both are fully incorporated.

Pour the mixture into an airtight container and refrigerate for 6 hours or for up to 1 month.

Yields: frosting for 24 cupcakes

For Your Nut-Free Kid

There are a lot of options if your child is allergic to nuts. Here are five healthy alternatives for sandwiches you may not have thought of:

- **Cream Cheese**—nice and thick, spreadable texture, and now available in a wide variety of flavors ranging from fruit to vegetable.
- **Guacamole**—a hearty sandwich topping, also goes especially well with pitas and tortillas.
- **Sunflower Butters**—made in dedicated facilities and specifically created for kids with peanut allergies or who might be attending peanut-free schools.
- **Hummus**—you can buy this garbanzo (and keep an eye out: sometimes sesame) spread or make your own. High in protein, it's especially good for vegetarians.
- **Veggie Purees**—easy to make in a blender or food processor, colorful and tasty.

If your child has tree nut or peanut allergies, you still have plenty of great-tasting, healthful, pleasing options. Take these Whoopie-Cookie pies, for example. (Who wouldn't?) After a Turkey "Aram" Roll Sandwich with Blueberry Salsa, or Lemony Chicken & Orzo Pasta Soup, they're yummy and make for one of the best desserts ever.

TURKEY "ARAM" ROLL SANDWICHES
WITH BLUEBERRY SALSA

Peanut-free, Tree-nut-free, and Wheat-free, too!
Prep Time: 15 minutes
Cook Time: none

½ **cup reduced-fat mayonnaise**
2 **teaspoons curry powder**
1 **pint blueberries**
1 **jalapeño pepper, seeded and chopped**
1 **kiwi, peeled and diced**
Juice of 1 lime
¼ **red onion, finely chopped**
½ **teaspoon salt**
8 **butter lettuce leaves**
4 **slices deli turkey**

For Mayo: Combine mayonnaise and curry powder in a bowl; stir until smooth.

For Salsa: Add blueberries, jalapeño, kiwi, lime juice, red onion, and salt in another bowl; gently fold to combine. Let salsa rest for 5 minutes for flavors to incorporate.

Top each lettuce leaf with 1 tablespoon mayo mixture, ½ slice deli turkey, and 1 tablespoon plus 1Ð teaspoons blueberry salsa. Roll up to serve.

Yields: 4 servings

LEMONY CHICKEN & ORZO PASTA SOUP

Prep Time: 15 minutes

Cook Time: 45 minutes

1 tablespoon olive oil

1 medium leek, white and pale-green parts only, halved lengthwise,
sliced crosswise ½-inch thick

1 celery stalk, sliced crosswise ½-inch thick

12 ounces skinless, boneless chicken thighs

6 cups low-sodium chicken broth

Kosher salt and freshly ground pepper

½ cup orzo

¼ cup chopped fresh dill

Lemon halves (optional, for serving)

Heat oil in a large heavy pot over medium heat.

Add leek and celery and cook, stirring often, until vegetables are
soft, 5 to 8 minutes.

Add chicken and broth; season with salt and pepper. Bring to a boil,
cover, reduce heat, and simmer until chicken is cooked through, 15
to 20 minutes.

Transfer chicken to a plate. Let cool, then shred chicken with two
forks into bite-size pieces.

Return broth to a boil. Add orzo and cook until al dente, 8 to 10
minutes.

Remove pot from heat. Stir in chicken and dill.

If desired, serve with lemon halves for squeezing over.

Yields: 4 servings

WHOOPIE-COOKIE PIES

Prep Time: 30 minutes
Cook Time: 1 hour

INGREDIENTS FOR WHOOPIE-COOKIES

2 cups all-purpose flour

½ cup your favorite Dutch cocoa powder (I suggest Droste—
produced in a dedicated nut-free facility)

1¼ teaspoons baking soda

1 teaspoon salt

1 cup well-shaken buttermilk

1 teaspoon vanilla

1 stick (½ cup) unsalted butter, softened

1 cup packed brown sugar

1 large egg

INGREDIENTS FOR FLUFFY FILLING

1 stick (½ cup) unsalted butter, softened

1¼ cups confectioners sugar

2 cups marshmallow fluff cream

1 teaspoon vanilla

Preheat oven to 350°F.

Whisk together flour, cocoa, baking soda, and salt in a bowl until combined. Stir together buttermilk and vanilla in a small bowl.

Beat together butter and brown sugar in a large bowl with an electric mixer at medium-high speed until pale and fluffy, about 3 minutes in a standing mixer or 5 minutes with a handheld mixer; then add egg, beating until combined well. Reduce speed to low and alternately mix in flour mixture and buttermilk in batches, beginning and ending with flour, scraping down sides of bowl occasionally, and mixing until smooth.

Spoon ¼-cup mounds of batter about 2 inches apart onto two buttered large baking sheets. Bake in upper and lower thirds of oven, switching position of sheets halfway through baking, until tops are puffed and cakes spring back when touched, 11 to 13 minutes. Transfer with a metal spatula to a rack to cool completely.

To make the Fluffy Filling: Beat together butter, confectioners sugar, marshmallow, and vanilla in a bowl with electric mixer at medium speed until smooth, about 3 minutes.

Assemble pies: Spread a rounded tablespoon of filling on flat sides of half of cakes and top with remaining cakes.

Yields: 8 individual pies

For Your Seafood-Free Kid

First things first: Nope, sushi does not have to mean "raw fish," and, yes, your kids will like it! Sushi actually means "sticky rice," and it has always fostered inventiveness, so feel free to add in chicken or beef, or even a plain, sliced omelet. The number of sushi fillings is virtually endless, making sushi a great activity, as well. A hearty curried chicken mimics tuna fish, and the big finish is a delish bento box dessert.

SEAFOOD-FREE SUSHI

Prep Time: 40 minutes

Cook Time: 2 minutes

3 cups sushi rice

3 cups water

3 tablespoons sushi vinegar

1 package precooked or preroasted nori sheets

1 bunch asparagus

1 bag carrot sticks or mini carrots

Optional add-ins: wasabi paste, grilled chicken or beef, sliced
    omelet

Measure 2 cups of sushi rice into a large bowl. Traditionally the rice is rinsed first by stirring it in cold water, carefully pouring off the cloudy, starch-filled water, and repeating twice.

Set in a colander to drain for about 30 minutes.

While the rice is draining, and later, while it is cooking, you can prepare little piles or stations for sushi assembly. Set out a bowl of water to keep hands moist while spreading rice. If using wasabi, put a few spoonfuls in a bowl for easy access and cover (and warn kids about how spicy it is!).

Cut sheets of nori in half, storing in a large zipper bag to keep moist.

Slice asparagus and carrot into strips about 1 inch in height.

Briefly steam asparagus and carrot either in a steamer over the stove or in a covered dish with a little water in the microwave on high. In either case, it should take about 2 minutes, depending on the thickness of the asparagus.

Arrange materials on and around a large cutting board, including water, wasabi, nori, vegetables, and rice. Place a sheet of nori a bamboo mat so that the length is parallel to the bamboo, wet your hands, and take about a cup of rice (you will quickly see why it is called *sticky rice* and why you need to keep your hands wet).

As you place the rice onto the nori sheet, fashion it into a long column that makes a strip right across the middle of the sheet. Gently press it toward the edges, so the whole sheet is covered with a thin blanket of rice, just a grain or two thick. Keep your fingers wet if necessary, but try to use as little water as possible to avoid dampening the rice.

If you're using wasabi, take a tiny dab of it on your finger and make an almost transparent green strip across the rice. Across the middle of the sheet, lay out an asparagus spear and enough carrot slivers to run the length of the roll.

To roll, gently take an edge of the mat in both hands, leaving it on the board or counter surface. Roll the mat and sheet together about one third of the way. Gently apply pressure and try to keep the roll rounded rather than flat.

Unroll slightly and repeat twice more, also at one-third intervals. By the end, the mat should have a substantial lip overlaying the roll, and that lip can be tucked under the roll so that the almost finished product is completely wrapped in bamboo. Now you can fine-tune the roll with pressure to make sure it is perfectly rounded.

Remove the mat and use your sharpest knife to cut the rolls into six or eight pieces, depending on how thick you want them. (Probably NOT a step for the kids.) To make sure the pieces are all even, first cut the roll in half and then cut each half evenly into two or three more pieces.

Repeat with remaining sheets, rice, and fillings until finished. Arrange on a plate or platter, and serve with shallow bowls of light soy sauce.

Yields: 12 sushi rolls

"MOCK" TUNA FISH (CURRIED CHICKEN SALAD) SANDWICH

Prep Time: 10 minutes

3 grilled chicken breasts (chopped)
2 stalks celery (chopped)
½ green apple (diced small)
¼ cup minced shallots
¼ cup golden raisins
¼ cup Greek yogurt
¼ cup mayonnaise
¼ teaspoon curry powder
Salt and pepper to taste

Combine all ingredients in bowl and blend well. Add additional mayonnaise to taste.

Serves: 6

Allergy-Free Bento Box

Bento boxes are beloved because the compartments help with portion control and naturally lead to a healthy variety of foods. You can find reasonably priced boxes at Target or order a special one online from Amazon.com. They can be filled with any favorite allergy-free dessert or just plain fruit. Each lunch is a little puzzle, an elegant surprise. And they don't have to take long to prepare.

Allergen-Free Candy Picks

Allergy-free certainly doesn't mean fun-free! Here are candies I've found to be free of the most common troublemakers, like peanuts, tree nuts, gluten, and dairy. Feel free to use these lists as general guidelines to help navigate your way down the grocery aisle. Remember, again, to check ingredient lists each and every time, as recipes and manufacturing practices change from time to time. Here are some all-time favorite, safe top-ten candies:

1. Airheads
2. Divvies
3. Dum Dums
4. Fun Dip
5. Life Savers (hard candies and gummies)
6. Nerds
7. Smarties
8. Starburst
9. Surf Sweets
10. Vermont Nut Free Chocolates

$$15$$

Baseline Advice
for Parents of
Food-Allergic Children

ALL OF THE ADVICE in this book distills into ten basic guidelines for being the parent of a food-allergic child.

We Must Protect and Serve Our Children

Sometimes parents are like policemen, and this familiar, venerable motto reinforces the aim and purpose of our role as parents. We remain mindful to not be perceived as food police in our quest to keep our children safe from their allergens, yet we must also adhere firmly to the *to protect and to serve* mantra. We must always remember that our children did not pick this path, and despite how difficult it is to maintain a safe perimeter, as parents we must lay aside our own fears and frustrations regarding food allergies and just serve in our role of parenting with empathy, compassion, and solid boundaries to raise independent citizens of the world—allergic or not.

In our lives, we must work with child care facilities to develop special care plans. We protect by always being on the lookout for hidden allergens in art supplies and bird feeders, in hand soaps and lotions, and everywhere in between. We serve by vigilantly ascertaining what is in each and every single food our children eat each and every time, and then we serve by being our most present selves and our most observant: to note if they respond to their meals with symptoms subtle or extreme, delayed or sudden. We are expert label readers and can bake up a decoy cupcake or whip up a birthday cake that could pass muster with flying colors on the Food Network. We seek to normalize our children's experiences by making sure that they blend in whenever possible and feel as normal as the next kid. We protect because in the most severe cases, our child's food allergies can quickly lead to anaphylaxis. We are at the ready to call 911 immediately, and we are prepared to protect by not hesitating to use our epinephrine auto-injectors, even if we are not 100 percent sure it is an allergic reaction, because as we serve our allergic children we understand that while it's scary to use the pen, it won't hurt our sons and daughters and instead could save a life.

We Maintain Strict Avoidance

Strict avoidance means everywhere: in the kitchen, in the bathroom, in the play areas, and beyond, every nook and every cranny, and then outward into the world at large. Treatment of a food allergy focuses largely on management of the medical condition. Right now there are no curative therapies for food allergy, so strict elimination of the offending food allergen and avoidance of any contact with it is the only way proven to avoid a reaction.

For our children, it's never okay to try a nibble or take a lick even just to see what it tastes like. This also means considering the possibility of potential exposures other than just eating the allergen, including through skin contact and inhalation of aerosolized allergens. Additional prophylactic measures like reading food labels each and every time, and then again at home, and one final time before serving—that's thrice—help ensure avoidance. Then there's exposure to trigger foods through cross-contamination or cross-contact. Don't assume: Always read food labels to make sure they don't contain an allergenic ingredient. Even if you think you know what's in a food, even if you have checked that particular brand before, check that label at the supermarket because ingredients and manufacturing facilities change from time to time. Avoidance also includes food ingredients that may be components of nonfood items like medications or vaccines. Allergen exposure lurks in many locations: lotions, soaps, cosmetics, children's board books, and art supplies. Even avoidance of saliva: This tenet includes strict avoidance and safe methods of kissing and sharing of meals and utensils.

Despite a world of temptation seemingly everywhere in life, this is good discipline for younger children, especially, to teach themselves to moderate, pay attention, and be mindful of their own health and best interests.

We Carry Our Own Medication

Even with avoidance measures and a seemingly constant observation of all the food surrounding our children, accidental inadvertent allergic reactions may well occur at any time—even when you least expect it. Unfortunately, despite best efforts and practices, being diligent with strict avoidance isn't always enough on its own. Sometimes your child can encounter a food allergy trigger even when you're all doing everything you can to avoid them. So while it's important for parents to have access to their epinephrine auto-injectors and accompanying rescue medication at all times, at the earliest opportunity and depending on your child's maturity and competency, your son or daughter must—*must*—be taught to carry his or her own medical bag, including two single-dose auto-injectors at school, at camp, and during activities.

There are plentiful lines of allergy apparel available online, ranging from epinephrine carrying cases to T-shirts to hoodies with epi-pockets to hold two standard-size auto-injectors. This useful gear is clearly labeled for your child's meds and includes information inserts for your child's name, emergency contact, and medical information.

The Centers for Disease Control and Prevention noted that "food allergies are a particular concern in the school environment." With nearly six million American children at risk of anaphylaxis, this is just one of the harsh realities of a successful food-allergic life. Granted, it's a huge emotional burden on our youngsters (and scary for them), but it is an important step toward self-empowerment to succeed in a confident food-allergic life.

We Refuse to Lie to Our Children

It is essential not to lie to children about their food allergies. As terrifying as the outcome might be, when your child asks about the severity or mentions a story he or she heard about an unsettling allergic reaction in the news, take a deep breath and be honest. Your child might know if you are lying, and this could break down the trust irreparably. The food allergy family must remain a team to succeed, and honesty—including the darker side of food allergy reactions, even in the worst case of fatalities—is an integral part of this teamwork.

Timing is everything, but do tell all the facts clearly and concisely and acknowledge that food allergies can be life-threatening. The unfortunate aspect about any type of deception is that when a child knows the truth and when parents contradict the knowledge, the child ends up doubting himself or herself. When parents tell children that what they know to be true in fact is not, they cause their children to choose between trusting themselves and trusting their parents. This is not a choice a child can make and remain intact and healthy. Researchers at Massachusetts Institute of Technology have found that children are not gullible and can in fact sense when parents are lying to them, causing them to distrust the very people who are their caretakers. Children also know when parents are withholding information.

When the stakes are so high with food allergy safety, we as parents need to accept that marginalizing this medical condition doesn't protect our children and that lying only leaves our sons and daughters knowing the truth and wondering why parents are lying about it. It's better to acknowledge problems and address them head-on rather than present a charade that is transparent and false.

Parents can tell the truth about negative events without focusing on the ugly details, and it's more reassuring for you to admit the situation in terms your children can grasp and talk through their feelings about it while they process the hard reality: Food allergies can be fatal. Then reinforce that your family has a comprehensive Food Allergy Action Plan firmly in place to manage the situation and that scientists and doctors are hard at work trying to figure out new ways to prevent and find a cure for food allergies—and are already broadening and deepening their

194

understanding of how to find a speedy and effective solution. Mostly, though, your child's understanding of the role he or she plays in his or her own health is imperative, and that's the straight truth of the matter.

We Refuse to Lie to Ourselves

Admit that we feel the terror, as well, and worry about the worst possible outcome ourselves. It's okay to cry, to feel angry, and to feel powerless and frustrated about this medical condition that has attacked your child's immune system and that at its worst could take your child away from you cruelly and without warning. Digesting the diagnosis of your child's food allergies disease can bring a flood of emotions. Some parents experience feelings of guilt and shame. I did, blaming myself and my darned DNA for my daughter's food allergies. Fear and grief are other common reactions to chronic illness. You may feel you're on a roller coaster of emotion—accepting one day and angry the next. It may help to remind yourself that these feelings are normal and will likely ease with time as you all adjust to a food-allergic lifestyle that suits your family.

How can you actively face the truth? A good place to start is by writing down all of your questions and taking them to your child's pediatrician and allergist to discuss one-on-one. Ask your child's doctor what specific steps you can take to optimize your son's or daughter's health. Accurate knowledge and straight talk without your child present at this meeting can help you feel empowered and reinvigorated. Also try to manage the elements in your family food allergy life that are within your control. Of course, you will not be able to regulate certain aspects of your child's food allergies, but you can choose to prepare allergy-safe meals, ensure all rescue medications are readily available and up to date, and build a strong support network you can rely upon and communicate with them about how they can best help you when you are struggling with the harsh truths about food allergies.

We Find Quiet Sources of Support
Away from Little Eyes

Let's face it, this medical condition can be too massive to contend with on our own. There is a wellspring of support out there nowadays, ranging from books to community groups to private therapists who specialize in stress management and chronic medical conditions. Having a good source of information and the opportunity to discuss food allergies with other families who share your concerns can be very helpful because they are dealing with the same challenges. A number of Internet sites and nonprofit organizations offer information and forums for discussing food allergies, and most are specifically for parents of children with food allergies. As you navigate this diagnosis, now more than ever, it's important to surround yourself with positive and supportive people so you can have a space to deal directly with the truth. Today there is awareness and a listening ear for your valid concerns and fears, a robust food allergy community alongside you to cheer you on in the day's hurdles and successes. Take advantage of it!

If you need to, minimize stress by letting go of unnecessary obligations for a while. You may be able to take time off from volunteer commitments, for instance, or ask for more help from family and friends. Furthermore, illness can be stressful for your entire family. It's not unusual for couples to experience strain on their relationship, so try to see things from the other's perspective and keep the lines of communication open to encourage support- ive dialogue. Make sure to plan for some alone time with your partner. Also encourage your partner to make time to care for himself or herself, especially if he or she is your child's primary caregiver.

We Make Mealtimes a Celebration of Food and Life

We want our children to grow up not fearing food. Yes, they need to avoid their allergen and become food label experts—home chef, even—but a mealtime is about so much more than just strapping on the feed bag and consuming mass quantities for nourishment and sustainability. Regardless of your nuclear makeup, the family table is a place to share the day's experiences, to bond together, to laugh, to meditate and reflect together, to acknowledge each other at the end of a busy day and check in.

Having a child with allergies does not have to negatively affect family mealtime. In fact, it can be a learning experience for all. Explore safe and alternative food choices, discover new reci- pes in books or on cooking channels and online, and be cre- ative. Your family may consider meeting with a registered dietitian specializing in food allergies to guide you through this process as you get started when the diagnosis is fresh to develop a stress- free, tailored feeding plan that includes a variety of safe, healthy, and delicious foods. If your child was already a picky eater, keep in mind that early childhood is the optimal time to expose your child to a wide variety of flavors and textures to encourage accep- tance of a variety of foods.

Even when a food allergy limits our children's diets, we have to make sure we don't limit that diet beyond what is necessary.

Children need time to get to know new foods, and a child who is served a limited variety of foods over and over again will learn to accept only those foods and will not be happy to have new foods served instead. So offering an allergy-safe new food and flavor alongside favorite foods is a good strategy. For children with food allergies, it is important to focus on the positive: This means all of the foods that are safe and delicious to try. Mealtime is the time for busy families to come together, so the atmosphere should always feel pleasant and relaxed. Children need role models with eating, and so the family meal is the ideal place to model appropriate mealtime behaviors and enjoyment of a variety of foods in a safe environment. Sharing stories and anecdotes from the day, describing the highlights and lowlights, and connecting with each other is all an integral part of the food sharing—so decide and commit to focus on that instead and eat together as a family.

We Do Not Play Favorites with Siblings in the Food-Allergic Household

Even immediately after a serious allergic reaction and/or scary hospitalization, be sure that you don't pour everything you have into the allergic child. It's useful to work together to cheer up your little patient and to celebrate a homecoming from the emergency room, but all of the other children are scared and traumatized as well, and the impact of bearing witness to anaphylaxis up close and personal leaves understandable—and usually short-term—emotional bruising and scars. Gently remember that siblings are as sad and powerless as you during this hospital stay, seek comfort from each other, and stay as balanced as humanly possible. When you can carve out time spent away from your child, try to find small things that you can enjoy and set realistic

198

short-term goals for yourself. Even small goals such as a visit to a park or museum or a phone call with a close friend can help you make the most of each day.

We Make Our Community Our Supporters

You never know who can help you out at school, on the playground, at basketball practice. Food allergy empathizers come in a wide variety of shapes and sizes, and often the ones you least expect step forward and link arms with you and your family! Be open to the curiosity and the inquiries—as nosy as some may be—as this is the first step toward an actual, real conversation. You set the tone with your attitude as you educate others. Sometimes annoying-sounding, probing questions can speedily lead to sharing information and supporting one another. Once there is a dialogue, you will find out what previous experiences others have had in managing food allergies. You may be disappointed that for some people a peanut butter and jelly sandwich is just a peanut butter and jelly sandwich and they have no method to imagine anything beyond that, but the truth is that you may also be pleasantly surprised. By remaining cool and collected, instead of initially overly emotional, you can establish a conversation with all ears on you, and then you can share the facts and experience of a trip to the hospital or your child's most recent allergic reaction very matter-of-factly. Communicating clearly and making the topic approachable can help make it indelible and will garner the best results for everyone involved. Every family's situation is unique, food allergies or not, and you may be surprised to find you can help each other cope with the many day-to-day aspects of managing family life and the stress that sometimes goes along with it.

We Dedicate Our Family to a
Non-Fear-Based Life

There isn't anything we can all do right now except to live well, avoid our allergens, carry our medication, think of innovative ways to tackle this problem, and hold on for a cure for food allergies; we need to keep spirits up. Besides, it's impossible to think clearly when our minds become flooded and overwhelmed with fear or anxiety. It's not unusual to feel anxious when you perceive there is a real threat to you or a loved one's safety, security, and welfare, and a good way to manage anxiety, or feelings of restlessness, worry, tension, and irritability, is by taking action. Anxiety can be useful in that it warns us of a very real threat, like a smoke alarm, and lets us know that we are at risk for danger. So to that extent, it's helpful to acknowledge this fear, but then you can banish it by making healthy choices that open you and your family to new experiences and learning.

Sometimes we panic, all of us, and one goal can be to help the mind get used to coping with panic, which takes the fear—of fear itself—away. One technique to reduce panic is to place the palm of your hand flat on your stomach and breathe slowly and deeply, inhaling and exhaling with your eyes closed. It can also help to visualize a happy place: Just take a moment to close your eyes and imagine a place of safety and calm. It could be a mental picture of you and your family walking on a beautiful beach or the entire gang snuggled up in bed with your little allergic one tucked in safe and sound right next to you. Or focus on a happy memory from your own childhood. Let the positive feelings soothe you until you begin to feel more relaxed.

Or try distracting yourselves from the worry—even just for fifteen minutes—by taking a family walk together around the block, making a cup of soothing tea, or taking a family yoga class.

Begin winding the family down an hour or two before family bedtimes and engage in calming activities such as listening to relaxing music or reading an enjoyable book together. Life is full of stresses, yet many of us feel that our lives must be perfect. Bad days and setbacks will always happen, and it's important to remember that life—allergic or not—is messy. It's our job as parents to provide our children with the education, encouragement, experience, and enthusiasm to get out into the world and safely live their lives to the fullest.

Conclusion

Dear World,

I need you to know that when I got pregnant, I was like a lot of you: It was dizzying and exhilarating, and I didn't know if I would succeed as a mother. I followed all of my obstetrician's rules and regulations and went for every prenatal visit; I stuck with the program.

You, world, don't walk in our food allergy mom shoes. We, food allergy mama bears, might seem a little cliquey, a little "helicoptery" for your liking and preference, a little neurotic to you who have less to worry about or even consider. You might find my attitudes at your child's birthday party to be annoying or pushy, and you might feel waves of indignation at how I seem to be nervously craning my neck, eyeballing and checking your child's plate of cookies. You had your own birth experience after all, your own trials and tribulations, no doubt. That's right, it's your child's lunchbox. So why am I trying to be all up in it?

"Stay out of activities," you may think or even say. Keep my kid over there. She can eat her own food, and that's my problem.

"Sorry," you say, "but what does the allergy have to do with me? I have my own problems. And you're just trying to control me and my kid. So back off." You might even snicker when you see me in the school hallway walking quickly with some pathetic-looking, clearly homemade medical bag, as I disappear into the school nurse's office. You might even whisper about me just a little, curiously, with the other mothers out in front of the preschool and then go awkwardly silent when I come out the door clutching my practice EpiPens and pretending I don't notice the silence.

Or, on the other hand, you may not. You may quietly observe me, silently thanking the universe that at least it isn't your child. You may think about me when you bake a birthday cake for the classroom and double-check the food label, maybe even by making a phone call to the 1-800 number on the box. You may—after much consideration and vacillating—invite us over to your house for a play date and spend hours before our first visit sanitizing and cleaning, recleaning, and checking labels, and then when I arrive, timid and terrified, with my child and step over your threshold, you may kindly and gently explain the steps you've taken, bring out the cookie wrappers for me to see for myself, sit me down with a hot cup of tea, and smile at me while our children whiz around your house.

You might imagine the relief I feel in that moment, the gratitude I can't even speak because it's so welled up in my throat that if I let it out, it wouldn't stop. You may discover that I'm not as alarmist as you thought, though the statistics are dismal and food allergies can be fatal. In time you might email me cheerful, silly jokes and distractions, or maybe you might work up the nerve to send me serious medical data you stumble upon on the Internet. You may decide that you really like me and defend me when another parent says something mean or insensitive on a field trip or at the school auction night. Later, you may choose to take responsibility for my child's allergen at your own home, so visits the kids spend together melt away into worry-free times for both our families.

We may all go for a swim together or take a family vacation trip, while you keep a silent vigil for my family and wish the best for us. You may pray for us someday. You may visit us in the hospital if my child has to be there for a lengthy time after a food allergy attack, bring us some comic books or stickers or a DVD. You should know that I have ridden in an ambulance with my child on a stretcher. You may cry for me sometimes when no one is around, and you probably intuitively know that of course I cry alone, too, when no one is around. You may rightly imagine that when you see the devastating news story that another child, someone else's—not mine—has succumbed to a food allergy at a camp or at school I have soberly witnessed the same news story.

There are words we parents don't usually say to each other, times when just a look or a hug or a triple-cleaned kitchen for a first visit are enough to say "I am your sister or brother" as we all make our way through this earthly experience side by side.

With gratitude, I thank you endlessly,
Mireille Schwartz

Glossary

504 Plan: Section 504 of the Rehabilitation Act of 1973, widely recognized as the first civil rights statute for persons with disabilities.

Allergen: A food or substance that triggers an allergic reaction.

Allergenic: A food or substance that has the properties to trigger an allergic reaction.

Allergic rhinitis: Commonly referred to as hay fever. The inflammation of the nasal passages caused by an allergic reaction to airborne substances.

Allergist: A doctor who specializes in the diagnosis, immunology, and treatment of allergies.

Allergy log: A comprehensive list of what the person eats for a period of time to determine what is causing a food allergy.

Allergy emergency kit: A durable, clearly marked bag containing injectable epinephrine, oral antihistamines, and written allergy information. Intended for true, IgE-mediated food allergies.

Anaphylaxis: An immediate, severe allergic reaction that causes difficulty breathing, swelling of the throat and tongue, and respiratory failure or shock due to a sudden drop in blood pressure. In extreme cases, it can be fatal.

Antihistamine: Medication used to block the effects of *histamine*, the chemical released during an allergic reaction. It does not stop the reaction but prevents the reaction from triggering some symptoms. It is available as both a prescription and an over-the-counter medication.

Asthma: A medical condition that causes narrowing of the small airways in the lungs, often arising from an allergic reaction. Symptoms include wheezing, coughing, chest tightness, and shortness of breath.

Auto-injector: Device that enables food-allergic individuals to inject themselves with a premeasured dose of *epinephrine* medication. It is available by prescription as EpiPen or Twinject, and now as AUVI-Q, a battery-powered compact epinephrine device that talks a user through the injection process step by step.

Avoidance: A food regimen designed to assist food-allergic individuals who must steer clear of any product that triggers reactions.

Benadryl (diphendydramine): A widely used *antihistamine* available in liquid, pill, or fastmelt/meltaway form. Very effective medication in treating food allergy reactions, but in the event of a severe allergic reaction, Benadryl may not be completely effective and *epinephrine* is required.

Biphasic allergic reaction: A second allergic reaction that occurs two to six hours after the first, often when the first wave of symptoms is under control.

Body integrity: A phrase coined by San Francisco Unified School District nurse Maryann Rainey, used to describe when teenagers become developmentally appropriate to manage their bodies themselves.

Casein (caseinate): A milk *protein*. Present in all *dairy* products.

Cross-contamination: This occurs when one food comes into contact with another food and their *proteins* mix, which is often invisible to the eye. Usually occurs when a safe food is manufactured on the same equipment as an unsafe food or when safe food is prepared or served with tainted utensils. Each food then contains small trace particles of the other food, which can trigger an allergic response.

Cytokines: Any of a number of substances that are secreted by specific cells of the immune system that carry signals locally between cells and thus have an effect on other cells.

Dairy: Containing or made from cow's milk, which is one of the most common allergenic foods.

Dedicated facility: A manufacturing facility that is free from a specific *allergen*. Because food is produced in a completely allergen-free environment, allergic individuals have the highest level of assurance that this food is safe to eat.

Eczema: An itchy and persistent red rash characterized by extreme dryness. The condition is commonly referred to as *atopic dermatitis*.

Elimination diet: Different foods and possible allergens are removed from one's environment until symptoms disappear. One by one, the substances are reintroduced until one triggers a reaction.

Enzyme: A substance that initiates the body's chemical reactions. *Food intolerances* can be caused by enzymatic defects in the digestive system because the body doesn't have the particular enzyme necessary to digest that food.

Eosinophilic esophagitis: Inflammation of the esophagus, an allergic inflammatory condition.

Epinephrine: Also known as adrenaline, a hormone and a neurotransmitter. Increases heart rate, contracts blood vessels, dilates air passages, and participates in the fight-or-flight response of the nervous system. It is available by prescription as EpiPen or Twinject and is your first and best defense in controlling severe allergy and/or anaphylactic reactions.

Fishy tomatoes: A hybrid of modified tomato plant that was being genetically engineered to resist frost using winter flounder fish.

Food allergen: A substance in a food, usually a *protein*, that triggers an allergic overreaction within the *immune system*.

Food allergy: A condition that results when the body's *immune system* mistakenly identifies a particular food as harmful. The body then creates antibodies to that particular food and in turn releases histamine chemicals that cause symptoms of allergic reaction.

Food diary: A log to track and report any recurring patterns in one's meals. Very useful in identifying a food allergy.

Gluten: *Protein* in wheat and other grains (including barley, rye, oats) that commonly triggers reactions in those with celiac disease.

GMOs: Foods produced from organisms that have had specific changes introduced into their DNA using the methods of genetic engineering.

Golden Gate Bridge: A suspension bridge spanning the Golden Gate strait, the mile-wide three-mile-long channel between San Francisco Bay and the Pacific Ocean. One of the most internationally recognized symbols of San Francisco, California, and the United States.

Heredity: The passing on of physical or mental characteristics genetically from one generation to another.

Histamine: A chemical released by the body during an allergic reaction; the cause of many of the symptoms of an allergic reaction.

Hives: Multiple red, raised, itchy bumps that form on the skin, often as the result of an allergic reaction. They can appear anywhere on the body.

Hygiene hypothesis: Empirically states that a lack of early childhood exposure to infectious agents, symbiotic microorganisms, and parasites increases susceptibility to allergic diseases by suppressing natural development of the immune system.

IgE antibodies: Immunoglobulin E. One of the antibodies that the *immune system* releases during an overreaction to an allergenic food. *Allergists* use a blood test to determine the presence of IgE to diagnose or rule out an allergy to a particular substance.

Immune system: The system that protects your body from diseases and infections. When a person has *food allergies*, the *immune system* identifies one or more foods as harmful.

Microbiota hypothesis: Emerging theory that low diversity of gut and stomach microbiota may be linked to allergic disease.

Oral immunotherapy: Also referred to as the "food challenge." A *food allergy* test that consists of a patient consuming the food he or she is suspected of being allergic to under a qualified doctor's close supervision, in a medical facility, with emergency medications and equipment readily available.

Placebo: A substance that has no therapeutic effect but is used as a control in testing new drugs or clinical trials.

Protein: A long chain of amino acids present throughout the body and in food. Foods that cause allergic reactions commonly contain proteins that the immune system mistakenly identifies as dangerous.

RAST: Radioallergosorbent test. A blood test that helps diagnose the presence of *IgE antibodies* in a patient to specific foods. Used by a doctor to identify or rule out particular food allergies.

REM sleep: A kind of sleep that occurs at intervals during the night and is characterized by rapid eye movements, more dreaming and bodily movement, and faster pulse and breathing.

Skin test: A *food allergy* test in which suspected *allergens* are injected in small amounts below the top layer of skin to determine whether the body reacts to the substance.

Synaptic pruning: A phrase coined by Yale psychiatrist Dr. Michel Jean-Baptise to describe the process of brain cells decreasing when a teenager turns around fifteen or sixteen years old.

Wheal: A small, raised swelling on the skin, as from an allergy prick test or an insect bite, that usually itches or burns. An overt sign of allergy.

XOLAIR (omalizumab): A prescription medication. Humanized antibody used to reduce sensitivity to inhaled or ingested allergens, especially in the control of moderate to severe allergic asthma that does not respond to high doses of corticosteroids.

Yoga: A stress-relieving system of exercises that combines physical and mental strength-building postures.

Acknowledgments

With gratitude to my wonderful family: my daughter Charlotte Jude Schwartz; my father; my beloved late grandparents, Sylvestre and Italia; Andrew and Renee and Bill and Debby and Barbara and the entire Schwartz family; baby Matthew Castro Jr.; Erik Noonan, Lynda and George Noonan, and Cathy Noonan. Special thanks to savvy, brilliant AMACOM Executive Editor Ellen Kadin, who has worked tirelessly to help this book from concept to shelf, mentored me in all aspects of book publishing, and provided tremendous camaraderie as well. Ellen: From the start, when I first reached out to you, you were welcoming, willing to listen, and a complete and total straight shooter. Every single dealing I've ever had with you has been a learning experience, and you have been remarkably patient as you explained even the rudimentary publishing basics to me. I'm beyond grateful. Thank you to my extraordinary editor Jennifer Holder, who gave the book "bones," as she dubbed them. She is amazing.

Thank you, Dr. Michel Jean-Baptiste and Plum and Lai, FARE, nurse Maryann Rainey, Andrew Ishibashi, Holly Giles, nurse Victoria Campagno, and Sophie Abitbol. Also, to my Canadian colleagues Gwen Smith, food allergy advocate and musician Kyle Dine, and children's book author Michelle Nel: Merci. Thank you to food allergy friends Billy Barnett and his family, Dennis Criteser, Cole Berggren, and Blue Bear School of Music. Thank you, Kevin Lyman and Sierra Lyman and 4Fini, for incredible kindness and support, and bottomless thanks to Dr. Anne Fox and her daughter Ruby Ida Fox.

About the Author

Mireille Schwartz lives with her family in San Francisco and is allergic to fish. She was featured in the 2013 Discovery Channel documentary *Food Allergies in America: An Emerging Epidemic*, narrated by food allergy parent and movie actor Steve Carell. The recipient of many awards, including a 2009 California State Senate Award for commitment to raising awareness, education, and advocacy on food allergy and anaphylaxis, Mireille Schwartz is CEO and founder of the Bay Area Allergy Advisory Board, established in 2007. The board's mission is to promote education and awareness and provide no-cost medical care and medication to Bay Area families with severely allergic children. She was a member of the board of directors for FAAN, now Food Allergy Research & Education (FARE), from 2009 until 2011 and is currently a 2016 to 2019 leader of FARE's Community Engagement Council. Mireille is an expert contributor to CNN Health, National Public Radio, Yahoo! News, and ABC7 News and a featured "Adult Allergies" columnist in *Allergic Living* magazine.

Index